Food Poisoning and Food Hygiene

Food Poisoning and Food Hygiene

Betty C. Hobbs
O.St.J., D.Sc., Ph.D., F.R.C.Path.,
Dip.Bact., F.R.S.H.

Food Hygiene Laboratory
Central Public Health Laboratory
London

Third Edition

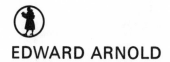

EDWARD ARNOLD

© Betty C. Hobbs 1974

First published 1953
by Edward Arnold (Publishers) Ltd.
25 Hill Street, London W1X 8LL

Second Edition 1968
Reprinted 1970
Third edition 1974
Reprinted 1975, 1976

Boards edition ISBN: 0 7131 4216 2
Paper edition   ISBN: 0 7131 4217 0

*Printed in Great Britain by
William Clowes & Sons Limited
London, Colchester and Beccles*

Preface to the Third Edition

The aim of this book, as outlined in the preface to the first edition, is to bring essential facts about food poisoning and its prevention to everyone engaged in food processing whether they are working in kitchens, shops or factories. The text is composed for those who teach the principles which govern the prevention of food poisoning, the local authority health officers, canteen supervisors, the managerial staff of food stores and factories and teachers in schools of catering and domestic science.

The facts are derived from the practical experience and knowledge gained by many workers in the field of public health during the past century. The method of presentation has been influenced by more recent experience gained in efforts to interest the food-handling public in a technical subject which should be so much their concern.

When the second edition was written there was evidence to show that many common foodstuffs both imported and home-produced are contaminated with food poisoning organisms, particularly those of the salmonella group, because the animals and birds providing these foods are hosts of the organisms. As the third edition is written there is no doubt that when animals and birds reared for human consumption are excreting salmonellae the food they provide may be contaminated with salmonellae also; the surfaces and equipment used for preparation and the hands of those working with the raw materials may convey the organisms almost immediately to other foods both cooked and uncooked. The function of food hygiene, therefore, is not only to prevent the spread of infection directly from the human carrier to food but also to prevent the spread of contamination in the kitchen, shop, factory and abattoir and especially to prevent organisms passing from raw to cooked foods. The chain of infection from animal to food to man needs greater emphasis in teaching. Food handlers can be infected from the foods they handle and become symptomless excreters or even clinical cases. Whereas legislation laid down in the various food laws will help to safeguard processed food against infection there is little effort made to protect the consumer or food worker against salmonellae in raw meat and poultry products.

The transference of infection from live animals and poultry to food is considered in relation to kitchens and shops under the Food Hygiene (General) Regulations, 1970 [Statutory Instruments No. 1172, HMSO], but families, farm, market and abattoir workers are susceptible to infection from many domestic animals and birds.

The number of incidents of food poisoning recorded annually have not altered significantly since the second edition, in fact they have risen slightly. The increase appears in sporadic cases and outbreaks due to the salmonella organisms. Yet, incidents due to the commonest serotype, *Salmonella typhimurium*, have declined while those due to many other serotypes have risen. Feedstuffs for animals both imported and home-produced are known to be a source of salmonellae which when fed to animals initiate the train of infection already described.

Since 1953 *Clostridium welchii* food poisoning has been fully recognized as a common cause of food poisoning. Outbreaks continue to occur without much improvement in the level of incidence. There are still too few kitchens with facilities designed specially for the rapid cooling of masses of cooked meat and poultry and with adequate cold storage space for larger bulks of cooked foods. A clear understanding of the necessity for quick cooling, cold storage and of the danger of leaving food at warm ambient temperatures is required.

Little more is known about food-borne virus infection than hitherto, but techniques for the isolation of viruses from foods have improved. Poliomyelitis and viral hepatitis have been traced to water and foods so that many other human and animal-borne viruses may be assumed to play a part in gastro-enteritis. Much bacterial food poisoning can be prevented by limiting the number of organisms in food by refrigeration; a virus would not grow in food but cause infection by viral particles passed from source to victim by means of food.

Outbreaks of *Vibrio parahaemolyticus* food poisoning are now recognized in countries other than Japan, including the United Kingdom, and the hazards of food poisoning from foods prepared in far-away flight kitchens are obvious when sick passengers arrive. Imported foods may introduce vibrios as well as salmonellae. *Bacillus cereus* long described as an agent of food poisoning in Scandinavia and eastern Europe is now recognized as a cause of food poisoning in the United Kingdom; it is known to produce toxin in cooked rice and perhaps other cereal products stored for some hours, without refrigeration, in the kitchen.

The realization has come slowly that *Escherichia coli* long known to be enteropathogenic for infants can also infect adults when certain strains are consumed in water and food. Perhaps Koch's postulates will be fulfilled for other microorganisms in the years to come, and we are still a long way from the full story of the danger from mycotoxins.

Accidental contamination of food with pesticide materials used for home and agricultural pests is rare in these countries but more common in the middle and far east. Careful legislation is necessary to protect man and his animals from these substances.

There is much talk about microbiological standards for all kinds of food. Used wisely, carefully chosen standards can help to improve the microbiological condition of foods so that spoilage and health hazards are reduced or eliminated. Standards which are too detailed and applied on a strictly legislative basis may be impossible to implement and therefore of little value.

We have missed the kindly guidance of Mr. L. Kluth whose consistent help was so much a part of the first and second editions; we regret that he died in September 1968. I thank Mr. R. J. Govett, Environmental Health and Technical Services Officer, London Borough of Brent for undertaking the revision of Chapters 14, 15 and 16.

The inspiration and help of the late Professor Robert Cruick-shank, of Sir Graham Wilson, Miss M. Barry and the late Lt.-Col. H. J. Bensted during the writing of the first and second editions will always be appreciated and I am thankful for their practical encouragement. Mr. W. Clifford's illustrations and photographs have contributed much to the interest of the book; we thank him and Mr. J. Gibson also for some more recent photographs.

I am grateful to Mrs. Isobel M. Maurer for the chapter on Disinfection and Sterilization and for editing help, and also to Miss Catherine F. Scott, School Meals Organizer, North Riding of Yorkshire and the late Miss Irene J. Martin, Domestic Science organizer the North Riding of Yorkshire for designing the lecture notes in the Appendix; they are used for short courses on Food Hygiene given to those working in the School Meals Service. The St. John Ambulance Association have generously allowed us to include the lecture notes which in their original form appeared in *Hygienic Food Handling* published by St. John Ambulance Association.

The following firms have submitted new or additional photographs:

The Hobart Manufacturing Co., Ltd., Leeds; James Stott & Co. (Engrs) Ltd., Leeds; MacFisheries Ltd., London; Waitrose, Food Group of the John Lewis Partnership.

We remember with gratitude those who contributed to the first and second editions:

Bowater-Scott Corporation Ltd., London; British Railways Board; Combined Laundry Group, London; Dawson Bros. Ltd., Woodford Green, Essex; Euk Catering Machinery Ltd., Oldham; Express Dairy Co. Ltd., London; The Gas Council; Hoover Ltd., Greenford, Middlesex; Mr. A. C. Horne, Chief Health Inspector, Hemel Hempstead; Jeyes' Sanitary Compounds Co. Ltd., Chigwell, Essex; King Edward's Hospital Fund for London; MacFisheries Ltd., London; Marks & Spencer Ltd.; Moorwood-Vulcan Ltd., Sheffield; Moreton Engineering Co. Ltd., Moreton-in-Wirral, Cheshire; The Chief Constable, York and North East Yorkshire Police; Pressarts Ltd., Leicester; Quiz Electrics Ltd., Teddington, Middlesex; J. Sainsbury Ltd., London; Staines Kitchen Equipment Co. Ltd., London; James Stott & Co. (Engineers) Ltd., Oldham; Mrs. E. Vernon, Central Public Health Laboratory, Colindale, London; T. Wall & Sons (Ice Cream) Ltd., London.

Neither the first, second or third editions would have been published without the faithful and thorough work of Miss Nancy Cockman who has compiled successive scripts, tables, figures and charts with her usual patience and fortitude, I am particularly grateful to her.

London, 1973   BCH

Contents

PART 1

Food Poisoning and Food-borne Infection

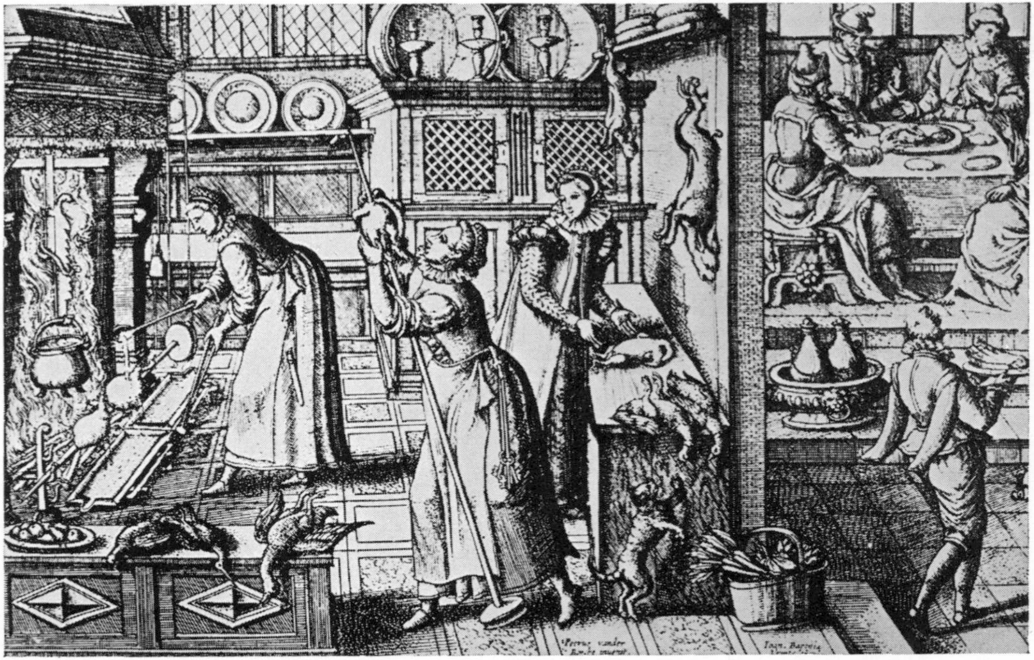

Fig. 1.　Ancient kitchen

1
Introduction

Food hygiene is a subject of wide scope. It aims to study methods for the production, preparation and presentation of food which is safe and of good keeping quality. It covers not only the proper handling of every variety of foodstuff and drink, and all the utensils and apparatus used in their preparation, service and consumption, but also the care and treatment of foods known to be contaminated with food-poisoning bacteria which have originated from the animal host supplying the food.

Food should be nourishing and attractive. It must be visibly clean and it must also be free from noxious materials. These harmful substances may be poisonous chemicals and even chemicals harmless in small amounts but damaging in large quantities. They may enter the food accidentally during growth, cultivation or preparation, accumulate in the food during storage in metal containers, form in the food through interaction of chemical components or they may be concentrated from the natural components of the food. Micro-organisms or germs may be introduced directly from infected food animals, or from workers, other foods or the environment during the preparation of foods. Poisonous substances may be produced by the growth of bacteria and moulds in food.

This book has been written for those engaged in food handling, with the purpose of explaining simply, in so far as our knowledge permits, what these various dangers are, how they arise, and how some of them can be prevented.

Noxious substances in food give rise to illness called food poisoning or gastroenteritis, which is usually characterized by vomiting and/or diarrhoea, and various abdominal disturbances. Food poisoning is no new disease, it has been recognized throughout the ages. Centuries ago the laws of the Israelites contained detailed information on foods to be eaten and foods to be abhorred, as well as on their methods of preparation and the cleanliness of the hands of the consumers. About 2000 BC, as recorded in the Book of Leviticus, Moses not only made many laws which protected his people against the ravages of infectious disease but also laid down rules about the washing of hands after killing animals for sacrifices and before eating. Many of these rules were based on a practical knowledge of personal hygiene and the necessity for cleanliness of those suffering from certain diseases.

Prohibited foods were those from scavenger animals, birds and fish such as pigs, vultures, ducks and mackerel. We know that pigs and ducks are natural excreters of salmonellae.

The accounts of food poisoning recorded in ancient history have generally been associated with chemical poisons—more especially with those deliberately introduced—but this is undoubtedly due to the fact that our knowledge of non-chemical, that is bacterial food poisoning, dates back no further than the latter part of the nineteenth century. Indeed the term ptomaine, i.e. alkaloid, poisoning was often used and may still be seen in the popular press to describe an outbreak of food poisoning which we know to have been caused by pathogenic or disease-producing micro-organisms or germs. The ptomaines are basic chemical substances formed by the breakdown or digestion of putrefying tissues; they were previously thought to be poisons formed in tainted foods, as food poisoning was assumed to be associated with taint. Now we know that foods heavily contaminated with food-poisoning germs may be normal in appearance, odour and taste.

There are some naturally occurring substances in plant life, such as deadly nightshade and toadstools, which can cause illness if consumed; also food may become contaminated during its preparation, with arsenic, zinc, copper, tin or other heavy metals, or with pesticides or disinfectants, with disastrous results. The amount of food poisoning due to these natural or chemical poisons is, however, small and it is not intended to enlarge on this subject. Nearly all our food poisoning is caused by the contamination of food by germs, the majority of which can grow actively in the food.

The study of micro-organisms including those known to cause disease is called (a) bacteriology, from the Greek word 'bactron', a rod, because the first germs observed through a microscope were tiny straight rods, or (b) virology, viruses being the smallest known micro-organisms. Bacteria, germs, microbes, micro-organisms, or simply organisms as they are variously called—and all these names will be used interchangeably in this book—were first seen and described in 1675 by a man who was not a professional scientist. van Leeuwenhoek was a linen draper in the town of Delft in

Holland but he was also an enthusiastic maker of lenses and magnifying apparatus. It was his hobby to examine objects of nature through the lenses which he mounted together to form a primitive microscope. One day, looking through his microscope at a drop of pond water, he saw not only a number of tiny animalcules but also tiny rods, many of which moved about actively within the microscope field. He described their size as one thousand times smaller than the eye of a louse. Next he took scrapings from his own teeth and, placing them under the microscope, he saw similar objects to those he found in the water. His drawings leave no doubt that these were the first bacteria to be described, but the significance of his findings was not appreciated at the time. Indeed, it was not until Louis Pasteur, the great French chemist and bacteriologist, demonstrated the essential part that bacteria played in fermentation processes in relation to wines and beers that the scientific world understood the significance of van Leeuwenhoek's observations made nearly 200 years before.

Pasteur developed methods of growing bacteria so that a more intimate study of them could be made. After his work on fermentation he turned his attention to the silkworm plague which was threatening to ruin the silk trade, then of paramount importance in France. He showed that the disease was caused by a bacterial infection of the silkworm and he was able to suggest successful measures for its control. After this he investigated diseases of animals and man, proving beyond doubt that bacteria were a necessary cause of many diseases. Pasteur's name will be forever associated with the dreadful disease, rabies, and the method he devised for its prevention, but another aspect of his work is of particular importance in the study of food hygiene. He was able to show clearly and completely that the old theory of spontaneous generation, that is life arising from the inanimate, was false. In other words, if a particular food product was sterilized by heat, living bacteria would not appear in the food unless they came from outside, from the air, from the hands, or from some other infected material.

About the same time Robert Koch was also making great discoveries in Germany; he found that anthrax, tuberculosis and cholera were caused by bacteria and he devised methods to grow these germs. From this time onwards the march of discovery in the field of bacteriology was rapid. From Europe, America, Japan and other parts of the world bacteriologists were fired with enthusiasm for their new science, and soon the causative microbes of gonorrhoea, erysipelas, diphtheria, typhoid fever, dysentery, plague, gangrene, boils, tetanus, scarlet fever and other illnesses had been found.

After thousands of years of darkness and superstition a great light was thrown on the cause of infection, and the door was opened for a vast study of the relation of bacteria to disease in animals and man. This study led to a knowledge of the way in which bacterial infections spread and, as a result, methods of prevention and of cure were found. Joseph Lister, applying the theories of Pasteur to surgery, discovered that wounds became septic by the action of bacteria. He introduced the use of antiseptics and disinfectants that would kill bacteria, and there was an immediate and astonishing reduction in wound sepsis.

Before 1850 the sanitary conditions in Britain were poor. From 1840 onwards began the Great Sanitary Awakening. Edwin Chadwick belonged to a family with a strong belief in personal cleanliness—a most unusual virtue in those days—and in 1842 he was instrumental in bringing out a *Report on the Sanitary Conditions of the Labouring Population of Great Britain*. The principle that environment influenced the physical and the mental well-being of the individual was introduced and, as the connection between filth and disease was gradually understood, measures were taken to control the disposal of sewage and the purity of water supplies.

In 1854 John Snow recognized that drinking water was concerned in the spread of cholera. William Budd in 1856 concluded that typhoid fever was spread by milk or water polluted by the excretion of an infected person. Prince Albert died of typhoid fever in 1861. In 1874 an outbreak of typhoid fever occurred in the Swiss town of Lauren and it was traced to polluted water; the result was that water supplies and sewage systems were redesigned to eliminate this danger. The chlorination of drinking water in Britain was initiated by Alexander Houston in 1905 during a typhoid epidemic in Lincoln, and its use has helped to abolish water-borne disease in this and other countries.

Toward the end of the nineteenth century the danger of infection by milk was discovered and in cities such as London, the heat treatment of milk by pasteurization began; this heat treatment kills many bacteria in the milk, including those that are harmful. The pasteurization of all supplies is not yet complete so that outbreaks of food poisoning and brucellosis still occur from tuberculin-tested raw milk and they will continue to do so until all milk is heat treated before distribution. The incidence of tuberculous infection in children drinking raw milk is now negligible in Great Britain, because most of the milk is pasteurized and also because the infection of cows has been almost eliminated by the destruction of animals found to be infected when subjected to the tuberculin test. A scheme for the eradication of brucellosis is in progress. A brief description of certain milk-borne and food-borne diseases is given in Chapter 8.

Acute poisoning and infection spread by food contaminated with disease-producing bacteria must have occurred from time immemorial, and they will continue to do so until we learn methods of control.

Drinking water is purified by sedimentation, filtration and chlorination; milk is heat treated and carefully packed in clean bottles or cartons; ice-cream is heat treated, cooled quickly and stored cold; liquid whole egg is heat treated (pasteurized), cooled quickly and frozen. Some foods are preserved by heat, cold, dehydration or chemicals before they reach the kitchen, but many of them are not. Raw foods can introduce food-poisoning organisms into kitchens and processed foods can be contaminated in the kitchen by other foods and by those preparing meals for consumption. To prevent the spread of infection by foodstuffs, therefore, we must either stop certain bacteria from entering food or, if they have entered unavoidably, make it impossible for growth to occur. When it is known that raw foods are consistently contaminated from animal or human sources they should be treated in some way before distribution to kill the particular food-poisoning organisms. At the same time, investigations should be made to find out how to produce such foods free from infection.

The first description of food poisoning bacteria was given by Dr. Gaertner in 1888; these bacteria were isolated from the organs of a man who had died from food poisoning during an outbreak in Germany affecting 59 other persons. Similar bacteria were found in the meat served to the victims, and also throughout the carcass from which the meat was cut. About the same time the so-called ptomaines, previously thought to cause food poisoning, were extracted from putrid foods and were found to be harmless if taken by mouth. These discoveries convinced many workers that the ptomaine theory of poisoning was wrong and, under the influence of Savage in the UK and Jordan in the United States, food poisoning gradually came to be associated with specific bacterial contamination.

In 1896 van Ermengem in Belgium described the organism, *Clostridium botulinum*, which is responsible for a very serious form of food poisoning known as botulism. *Cl. botulinum* produces in food a highly poisonous toxin affecting the nervous system and often causing death. Fortunately, botulism is rarely described in the United Kingdom, although it still occurs in other parts of the world.

In the years 1909 to 1923 many of the bacteria now known to be responsible for a large proportion of food poisoning incidents were grouped together under the generic name *Salmonella*, in honour of Dr. Salmon who isolated the first member of the group, the hog cholera bacillus, in 1885.

From 1914 onwards another group of bacteria, the staphylococci, were found to be concerned with food poisoning. Certain strains of staphylococci produce in food a poisonous substance or toxin which, if swallowed, gives rise to quick and violent reactions.

From 1945 to 1953, a fourth major causal agent of food poisoning was investigated and described, the anaerobic sporing bacillus *Cl. welchii*; this organism is similar to *Cl. botulinum* but the illness is usually mild with less disastrous results.

From time to time various common bacteria are thought to be responsible for food poisoning. They may be present in large numbers in the raw food or on surfaces or equipment, survive preparation or recontaminate the food after cooking.

The safety of food thus depends on freedom from the bacteria known to cause food poisoning and also from mass bacterial contamination usually resulting from careless storage. Clean food is free from visible dirt and bacterial spoilage; not all spoilage bacteria cause food poisoning and conversely the food-poisoning bacteria may not cause visible spoilage even when present in enormous numbers. The aim of food hygiene should be the production and service of food which is both safe and clean.

Under poor storage conditions bacteria can grow to large and dangerous numbers. Four main factors are important: (a) the initial safety of raw foods before their introduction into manufacturing establishments, shops, canteen and home kitchens, (b) the hygiene and care of those responsible for handling food during production and service, (c) the conditions under which food is stored, and (d) the general design and cleanliness of kitchens and equipment.

The incidence of food poisoning appeared to increase greatly after World War II; 7846 incidents were recorded in 1959. Table 1 gives the figures for 1961–1970. It may be asked why outbreaks of

TABLE 1. Recorded Food-poisoning Incidents* (England and Wales, 1961–1970)

Year	1961	1962	1963	1964	1965
Number of incidents	5,387	4,521	4,465	4,372	4,091

Year	1966	1967	1968	1969	1970
Number of incidents	3,744	4,256	5,084	6,436	6,107

* Outbreaks and sporadic cases.

food poisoning are still so common today when the standard of living is higher, when general or personal hygiene is improved and when knowledge is increasing. There are many answers to this question; they are partly related to the change in the way of life which began soon after the turn of the century. So insidious was the change that it was hardly noticed for several years, but in retrospect it can be dated to a period well before World War I, when food was cheap and for the most part tastes were simple. Thousands of the working population had, of necessity, to take their midday meal in some sort of eating-house. The majority of these were small, rather dingy places, often with underground basement kitchens with very inadequate washing and sanitary facilities; yet it was uncommon for intestinal infection to follow meals taken in such establishments. The cost of these meals was very cheap by present-day standards, and for the most part they were good simple meat meals, generally freshly roasted or boiled joints with vegetables, often with nothing to follow. At the slightly more expensive houses there would be a boiled pudding or fruit tart.

Although the standard of hygiene observed in these eating-houses might be lower than the level today, the chances of food poisoning following such meals were very small, because the simple meals were freshly cooked and quickly served to relatively small groups of consumers.

With the increased facilities the habits of people changed; the cinema became popular, motor transport increased and there were more attractive restaurants to meet a growing need. Immediately after World War I the popularity of large restaurants increased; they served food at reasonable prices but often pre-cooked. Made-up meat dishes and cream-filled cakes, prepared ahead of requirements and ideal for bacterial growth, became popular also. After World War II almost the whole nation participated in communal feeding, when in addition to the public restaurant, canteens were set up in factories, schools and offices. Although the habit of communal feeding had been growing for years the nation was entirely unprepared for this enormous change-over. Canteen kitchens, often converted in a hurry, were of unsuitable design and inadequate for the number of meals required. Kitchens originally intended for serving a certain number of meals were forced to provide double or even treble that number, sometimes with limited equipment and inadequate staff. At the same time few of the people in charge of these catering establishments had any knowledge of the precautions necessary for the preparation, cooking and serving of meals on this large scale.

Under such conditions it is not surprising that errors occurred in the bulk handling of food. Large numbers of persons were served from one canteen kitchen, and a single infected dish could affect many; whereas a similar incident in a small household would affect one or two persons only.

Another factor of importance was the growing import trade of protein foods needed to feed the increasing human and animal population. Egg products, meats, coconut and dried feeding stuffs for animals, all now known to contain food-poisoning organisms, were brought into the country in enormous quantities to be eaten raw, cooked or used in the bulk manufacture of many foods which were purchased more and more by the busy housewife with her family to feed and a job to do.

Other problems in Britain during and after World War II included shortages of certain foods and more particularly of meat. The housewife and the canteen supervisor acquired the habit of hoarding left-overs and cooking their small cuts of meat the day before required in order to slice them more economically when they were cold. Some of these habits have remained and provision for cold storage is still inadequate with only two-thirds of British households equipped with refrigeration.

From 1960 onwards, factory farming became popular and the production of foods, poultry and meat particularly, increased. Convenience foods helped the busy army of housewives working both inside and outside their homes.

In 1939, a public health bacteriological service was instituted
which supplemented the work of the public and private analysts.
The number of laboratories increased, and they provided more
facilities for the investigation of food-poisoning outbreaks. Also,
teaching on the subject of food hygiene became popular. In 1950,
for the first time, the combined recorded food-poisoning incidents
from the Public Health Laboratory Service and the Department
of Health and Social Security, which receives all notifications of
food poisoning from local authorities, were gathered together, so
that a great deal of information on food poisoning hitherto un-
recorded was brought to light. In 1955, legislation on food hygiene
was passed.

What are the aims, therefore, for personal hygiene, food storage,
the general design of kitchens and their equipment, and the safety of
basic food ingredients? First, it must be recognized that the natural
hosts of food-poisoning bacteria and viruses are the human and
animal body. Second, efforts should be made to reduce the rates
of excretion of salmonellae by animals and poultry by eliminating
salmonellae from feeding stuffs and by care in animal husbandry.
Third, essential raw food commodities known to be contaminated
with salmonellae should be rendered safe before distribution or
warnings given. Fourth, foods susceptible to bacterial growth
should be cooled quickly and kept cold after cooking. Fifth,
kitchens should be designed to provide conditions for well-ordered
working, with plenty of space, good ventilation and lighting, and
with equipment in good repair readily accessible and easily
dismantled for cleaning and disinfection. Sixth, kitchen staff should
be taught the principles of hygiene in relation to themselves, the
foods they handle and their surroundings and equipment.

Before considering these in greater detail it may be useful to
describe the shape, size, habits and requirements of those minute
organisms which cause disease and poison food—the bacteria.

2

Elementary Bacteriology

The size, shape and habits of bacteria

It is difficult to understand the chain of circumstances which must precede an outbreak of disease caused by contaminated food, without knowing something about the organisms responsible.

The characteristics of bacteria in relation to their source and reservoir and a knowledge of their ability to survive and grow in food are important factors in the control of both food poisoning and food spoilage. Prevention is much concerned with the destruction of bacteria and with the inhibition of growth.

Bacteria are minute, single-celled organisms of variable shape and activity. Along with the algae, fungi or moulds, and the lichens they are classified as the lowest forms of plant life. Bacteria are everywhere in soil, water, dust and in air. There are thousands of different types and many perform useful functions. Some turn decaying vegetable matter into manure; others, within the human or animal body, assist in the development of certain vitamins essential to health; some can be harnessed for fermentation processes such as in the production of beer or wine and the manufacture of cheese; and others are used to produce antibiotics for the cure of disease. Only a very small proportion of the total bacterial population are dangerous because they can cause disease in man and animals.

Bacteria are so small that individually they cannot be seen without a microscope. They may be as small as 1/2,000 mm and clusters of a thousand or more are only just visible to the naked eye. Fifty thousand placed side by side may measure barely an inch (25 mm). Seen under the high-powered lens of a microscope with a magnification of 500 to 1,000 times (Fig. 2), the bacteria which may be spread by food are round or rod shaped and appear in one or other of the following forms according to the type of organism. Some are mobile in fluids and swim about by means of hair-like processes which arise singly or in clusters from one end, both ends, or from all around the cells. Some possess capsules, outer mucinous coats which protect them against substances which might destroy them. Some can produce resting bodies

12

called spores (Fig. 2d) when conditions are unfavourable for growth, and particularly when there is a lack of moisture. These spores form within the bacterial cell which afterwards gradually

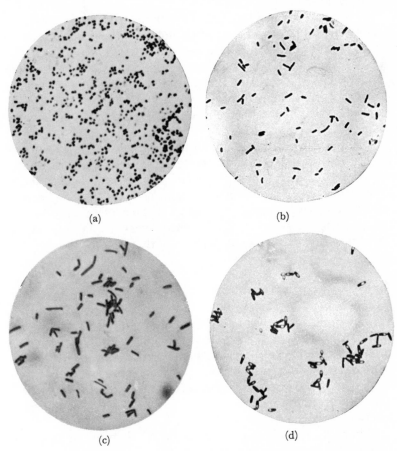

(a)

(b)

(c)

(d)

FIG. 2. Food-poisoning bacteria: (a) Staphylococcus; (b) Salmonella; (c) *Clostridium welchii*; (d) *Clostridium botulinum*—showing spores

disintegrates. Many can withstand high temperatures for long periods and the processes required for the sterilization of canned foods are based on the time and temperature calculated to destroy the most heat-resistant spores. Sporing bacteria, when allowed to multiply in foodstuffs, may be responsible for spoilage decomposing the food with gas production. A few species, for example *Clostridium welchii*, cause food poisoning when ingested in large numbers after multiplication in foods, particularly cooked meat dishes; *Clostridium botulinum*, the cause of botulism, produces a highly poisonous toxin while growing in food.

Although most food-poisoning bacteria cause symptoms only when eaten in large numbers after multiplication in food they do not usually alter the appearance, taste or smell of the food. The types of bacteria which break down protein so that there is visible spoilage leading to putrefaction detectable by smell do not usually cause food poisoning, although the early onset of obvious spoilage is a safeguard against the consumption of heavily contaminated foods.

It is generally impossible by visual inspection to know whether food is dangerously contaminated with food-poisoning organisms or not. Animals infected during life may reach the market or slaughterhouse excreting small numbers of food-poisoning bacteria yet without symptoms. Even in the early stages of illness there may be no obvious signs of changes in the carcass or offal to warn the meat inspector or veterinary surgeon of the potential danger.

Growth and multiplication

Bacteria multiply by simple division into two, and under suitable conditions of environment and temperature this occurs every 20 or 30 minutes. Thus one cell could become over 2 million in 7 hours and 7,000 million cells after 12 hours' continuous growth. When each cell has grown to its maximum size, a constriction appears at both sides of the centre axis, the outside membrane or envelope of the cell grows inwards and forms a division which finally splits, releasing two new twin cells (Fig. 3).

When the available nutrient has been exhausted or the waste products of growth make the environment unsuitable, for example, by the production of acid, growth ceases and the cell dies. The length of life of a bacterial cell varies according to the food or medium on or within which it is growing or resting, and also according to the type of organism. The spores produced by certain bacteria can survive in a dormant condition for long periods of time under adverse conditions but when suitable conditions of food, moisture and temperature return they are able to germinate into actively growing bacteria again.

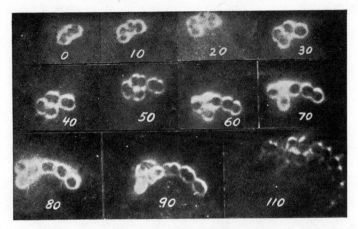

FIG. 3.   Division or multiplication of bacteria. (From G. Knaysi, 1951, *Elements of Bacterial Cytology*, Comstock, Ithaca, N.Y.)

Conditions for growth and multiplication of bacteria

In the laboratory a variety of media are made to suit the growth requirements of different types of bacteria. Most of them have a meat-broth base set into a firm gel by means of agar, a substance which is extracted from seaweed. Agar has special properties; it melts at a high temperature and sets at a low temperature and it is thus more suitable for bacterial media·than gelatin which melts at temperatures below those required for the growth of many bacteria. Blood, serum, milk or other protein matter may be added for enrichment.

When bacteria are spread on the surface of agar media in a petri dish and left overnight at a suitable temperature, such as 37 °C (98·6 °F)—blood heat—they start to grow. By division of each cell into two every 15–30 minutes a small heap of bacteria is formed consisting of millions of cells, which is called a colony. Every kind of bacterium has a typical colony form; the size, shape, colour and consistency of these colonies on particular culture media help in identification (Fig. 4). Another method by which we can identify the different types of bacteria, as well as by their appearance under the microscope and on the surface of agar media, is to observe their activity in liquid media containing different sugars. Some bacteria ferment certain sugars with the production of acid and gas, others ferment different ones, some produce acid only, while others produce neither acid nor gas. There are chemical tests, too, which are often useful for distinguishing between different bacteria.

The individual members of bacterial groups may be divisible also by serological methods. For example, the agglutination of organisms brought about by the altered blood serum of human beings or animals infected with the same organism may be used for this purpose.

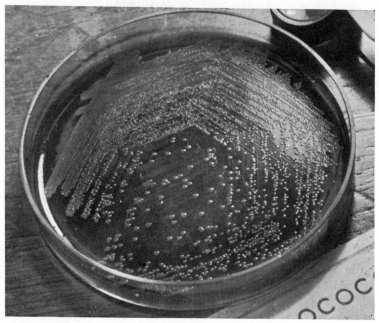

FIG. 4.   Colonies of staphylococci

An even finer differentiation into types is sometimes possible by means of bacteriophages, which are viruses parasitic on bacteria. The bacteria are identified according to the types of invading phage, which are specific to the bacterial host cell. Cultivated phages are inoculated on to bacterial cultures which they destroy. *Salmonella typhi*, some other salmonellae and staphylococci are typed in this way.

Many years of laboratory work have led to the development of special kinds of culture media which will enhance the growth of certain types of bacteria and depress other types. To isolate food-poisoning bacteria from foodstuffs there are media which will suppress the growth of harmless or non-pathogenic bacteria, and encourage harmful or pathogenic bacteria to grow.

Bacteria will live and multiply in many foodstuffs; sometimes the type of food and the atmospheric temperature and humidity of the

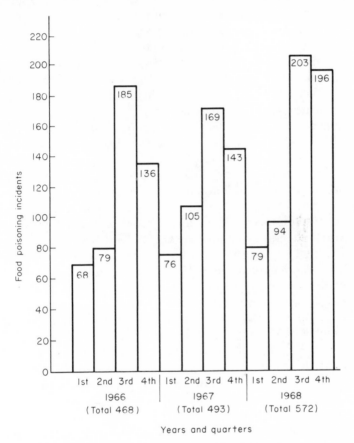

Fig. 5.   Seasonal prevalence of food poisoning

kitchen provide conditions similar to those used for cultivation in the laboratory. Meats and poultry are good examples: whether raw or cooked they are excellent media for bacterial growth; pies, stews and gravies resemble laboratory media. Milk and egg products, including custards and trifles, soft cheese and cream, are all good media for growth. Bacteria will multiply in these foods when they are stored in the shop or kitchen without refrigeration; in the same way, they multiply in specially prepared medium inoculated in the laboratory and incubated for warmth. Thus food poisoning occurs more frequently in the summer than in the winter (Fig. 5).

Most bacteria require air to live actively, but some can multiply only in the absence of oxygen; they are called anaerobes. Included in this group are the sporing organisms *Cl. welchii* causing food poisoning, and *Cl. botulinum* causing botulism. *Cl. welchii* flourishes under the conditions found in the centre of rolled joints of meat, in poultry carcasses and in boiled masses of meat such as beef, cut up or minced and in stews. Care must be taken to destroy the spores of bacilli when meat, vegetables and other foods are canned. Because adequate heat treatment may not be given in the home, amateur canning or bottling of meats and vegetables is discouraged.

Pathogenic or harmful organisms grow best at the temperature of the body, which is 37 °C (98·6 °F), although the majority will multiply between 15 and 45 °C (59 and 113 °F). Except for *Cl. welchii*, which grows well at temperatures up to 47 °C (117 °F) and even up to 50 °C (122 °F), the ability of most bacteria to multiply falls off rapidly above 45 °C (113 °F) and only a few groups can grow at temperatures above 50 °C (122 °F). Non-sporing cells of food-poisoning bacteria are killed at temperatures above 60 °C (140 °F), the length of time (10 to 30 minutes or more) required depending on the types of organisms (Fig. 6). For example, to make milk safe, i.e. free from harmful bacteria, it is pasteurized at 62·8 °C (145 °F) for 30 minutes, or at 71·7 °C (161 °F) for 15 seconds, or at higher temperatures for an even shorter time (Fig. 18), such as 132 °C (270 °F) for not less than 1 second as laid down in the Milk (Special Designation) (Amendment) Regulations 1965 for 'Ultra Heat Treated' milk. This milk must be put into sterile containers using aseptic precautions and is said to have a shelf life of several months.

Methods of heat treatment, e.g. pasteurization, can be applied to other foodstuffs such as fresh cream, imitation cream, ice-cream mix and liquid egg and albumen (see Chapter 5).

Boiling kills living cells, with the exception of spores, in a few seconds; however, spores may require to be boiled for 5 or more hours before they are killed. To destroy them in a shorter time, temperatures above boiling obtained by the use of steam under pressure, must be used. Figure 7 illustrates the effect of temperature on the vegetative cells of bacteria. The toxic substance produced by staphylococci in food needs boiling for 20 to 30 minutes before

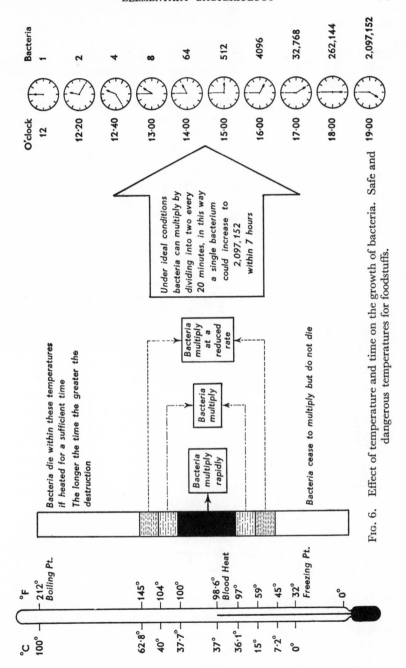

Fig. 6. Effect of temperature and time on the growth of bacteria. Safe and dangerous temperatures for foodstuffs.

it is destroyed, but the toxin of *Cl. botulinum* is destroyed more readily by heat.

Extreme cold will not kill all bacteria, but it will prevent them multiplying and for this reason foods which support bacterial growth should be stored at low temperatures. Domestic refrigerators not only delay the spoilage of foods but prevent the growth of harmful bacteria. Freezing kills a proportion of cells. Safety

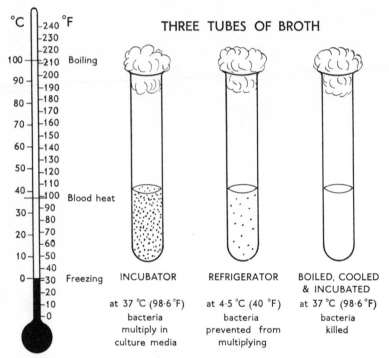

FIG. 7.   The effect of temperature on bacterial cells

measures for ice-cream include both heat treatment and cold storage with rapid cooling in between.

Bacteria cannot multiply without water. Cold cooked meats contain sufficient moisture to support growth, whereas in dehydrated products such as desiccated soup or milk powder bacteria will survive but remain dormant until there is sufficient water added to revive them.

The addition of various salts, acids and sugar to laboratory media is carefully controlled. The presence of these substances in varying amounts in different foodstuffs exerts an effect on the ability of organisms not only to grow but to survive.

The use of these substances as preservatives and the effect of antibiotics, irradiation and fumigation are discussed in Chapter 11.

Quite simply, bacteria are single-celled living organisms which are present almost everywhere, often in large numbers. Mostly they are harmless but some cause spoilage in foods and others give rise to disease in the human and animal body. Both humans and animals may harbour disease-producing pathogenic bacteria which may be passed to foodstuffs and multiply when conditions of temperature, time and moisture are suitable. These living bacterial cells will cease to multiply in the cold and die if they are too hot, although the structures known as spores, produced in some cells by certain bacteria, can survive long periods of boiling.

The next chapter describes the bacteria which cause food poisoning, particularly, where they live, their reservoirs, and their behaviour.

3
Bacterial Causes of Food Poisoning

Bacterial food poisoning is a disturbance of the gastrointestinal tract, with abdominal pain and diarrhoea and usually vomiting also. The onset may be any time between 2 and 48 hours—longer for botulism—after eating contaminated food. There are eight groups of bacteria which are known to cause food poisoning:

Salmonella	*Vibrio parahaemolyticus*
Staphylococcus	*Bacillus cereus*
Clostridium welchii	*Escherichia coli*
Clostridium botulinum	*Streptococcus*

The first three are common in many countries; *Vibrio parahaemolyticus* is the commonest form of food poisoning in Japan. *Clostridium botulinum* occurs occasionally mostly in the northern hemisphere. It is suspected that *Bacillus cereus* may be fairly common and that certain serotypes of *Escherichia coli* may cause diarrhoea in adults. Streptococci have been described as causal agents in some countries; other organisms are occasionally reported to be associated with food poisoning.

TABLE 2. Bacterial food poisoning: Incubation period and duration of illness

Cause of food poisoning	Incubation period (hours)	Duration
Salmonella (infection)	12–36	1–7 days
Staphylococcus (toxin in food)	2–6	6–24 hours
Clostridium welchii (toxin in intestine)	8–22	12–24 hours
Clostridium botulinum (toxin in food)	24–72	Death in 24 hours to 8 days or slow convalescence over 6–8 months
Vibrio parahaemolyticus (infection)	2–48 (15)	2–5 days
Bacillus cereus (toxin in food)	2–15	1–2 days
Escherichia coli (infection)	12–72	1–7 days
Streptococcus (toxin in food)	3–22 (12)	24–48 hours
Others (unknown)	?	?

The duration of illness is mostly short, from 1 to 3 days, but patients with salmonella infection may not feel well for 7 or more days.

Clinical details, incubation periods and information about the foods eaten, how they were cooked and the ingredients are helpful to those examining suspected material in the laboratory. When an investigation is delayed or specimens are not available, relevant and accurate information may be the only means by which the cause of an outbreak may be established.

The general characteristics of the various types of food poisoning are described in the following pages and are summarized in Table 2.

Salmonella

The salmonella group of organisms causes food poisoning by infection; that is, by invasion of the body. They reach food directly or indirectly from animal excreta at time of slaughter, from human excreta or water polluted by sewage; also, in the kitchen they may be transferred from raw to cooked foods by hands, surfaces, utensils and other equipment. Probably illness occurs only when the organisms are ingested in large numbers, so that a chance contamination of the food by a small number of bacilli may not be harmful. When they are allowed to multiply in the food, that is, if the lightly contaminated food stands for some hours in a warm room, then sufficient numbers of bacteria will develop to produce symptoms in the consumer.

The onset of illness occurs usually within 12 to 36 hours of eating the food, although the incubation period may be longer. The symptoms are characterized by fever, headache and general aching of the limbs, as well as by diarrhoea and vomiting. There may be 20 to 40 fatal cases each year mostly in infants, and elderly or sick people. The duration of illness is longer than that caused by the toxin of the staphylococcus and may be from 1 to 7 days. There are many hundreds of different types of salmonellae classified by serological methods and several types may be more finely divided by means of bacteriophage (see p. 16). The subdivisions are helpful for the investigation of outbreaks. All types can produce disease in man or animals.

Staphylococcus

Staphylococcal food poisoning follows the consumption of food heavily contaminated with certain types of *Staphylococcus aureus* which produce a poisonous or toxic substance in the food. Cooked foods such as meat and poultry intended to be eaten cold and prepared foods such as custards and trifles and creams also are readily contaminated by hands; the skin and nose frequently harbour staphylococci. Since the toxin is formed by the organism growing in food before it is eaten and not after it has entered the body, the incubation period may be as short as 2 hours but in general it is 4 to 6 hours. There is a rapid onset of symptoms characterized by severe vomiting, diarrhoea, abdominal pain and cramps, sometimes followed by collapse. Recovery is rapid.

Typing methods for staphylococci both by bacteriophage and serological methods have enabled the pathogenic species to be divided into groups, some of which are more common than others in food-poisoning incidents. There are several types of enterotoxin also which can be extracted from culture filtrates and foods and identified serologically. Human and animal feeding experiments have been used also. Whereas the staphylococcus itself is fairly readily destroyed by the heat of pasteurization and normal cooking procedures, the toxin is more resistant to heat: it is destroyed gradually during boiling for 30 minutes. It may remain active after light cooking.

Clostridium welchii

Organisms of the *Clostridium* group will grow only in the absence of oxygen and they are spore bearing. *Cl. welchii* is a common organism; it can survive, by means of hardy little spores, for long periods of time in dust and soil. It is frequently found in excreta from humans and animals and on raw meats, poultry and other foods including dehydrated products. Illness occurs after eating food, particularly meat, grossly contaminated with *Cl. welchii* which has multiplied during long slow cooling and storage of cooked meat and poultry, stews, pies or gravy in the kitchen or canteen. The spores vary in their ability to withstand heat. Some strains of *Cl. welchii* can survive hours of boiling; others only a few minutes. The spores may not be destroyed in boiled, stewed, steamed, braised or even roasted foods, particularly those cooked in bulk. After cooking, the spores readily germinate into bacteria which multiply rapidly under favourable conditions including temperatures up to 50°C (122°F); there is little growth below 15°C (59°F).

Symptoms occur from 8 to 22 hours after consuming the contaminated food; they include abdominal pain, diarrhoea and nausea but rarely vomiting; they may continue for 12 to 24 hours. The symptoms result from the activities of a large dose of organisms which form toxins in the intestine; an effective toxin is not formed in the food before it is eaten.

Two of the five types of *Cl. welchii*, classified according to their toxin production, are able to cause food-borne disease in man. Of these, type A is the more common agent of food poisoning, while type C causes a more serious condition called enteritis necroticans. Type C was first isolated from home-canned rabbit causing illness in Germany and it has been found in pork causing outbreaks in New Guinea. So far it has rarely been associated with human illness in the United Kingdom. The type A strains can be further divided into many serotypes by the use of specific antisera.

Clostridium botulinum

The toxin of *Cl. botulinum*, another anaerobic spore-bearing bacillus, is a highly poisonous substance produced as the organism grows in food. It affects the nervous system, causing an often fatal illness. Outbreaks and cases of botulism rarely occur in Great Britain but they are reported from other countries and depend on the feeding habits of the population (p. 61). The species is divided into six types according to the toxin produced; four are known to affect man. The spores are resistant to heat, and may survive boiling and even higher temperatures.

The toxin is sensitive to heat, and in pure form it is destroyed by boiling. Nevertheless, it may be protected when mixed with protein and other material in food. The toxin is lethal in very small doses and gives rise to symptoms quite different from those of the organisms just described. The incubation period varies from 24 hours or less to 72 hours, and the first signs of illness are lassitude, fatigue, headache and dizziness. Diarrhoea may be present at first but later the patient is obstinately constipated. The central nervous system becomes affected and there is a disturbance of vision; later, speech becomes difficult and there is paralysis of the throat muscles. The intoxication reaches its maximum within 24 hours to 8 days and death often occurs by paralysis of the respiratory centres. If, after 8 days, the patient survives, convalescence is slow. Life may be saved by giving antitoxin as soon as possible.

Bacillus cereus

Certain members of the *Bacillus* group which are commonly occurring aerobic spore-bearing organisms, and especially *B. cereus*, are known to cause food poisoning.

The spores of *B. cereus* are frequently present in cereals; they can survive light cooking and germinate into bacilli which grow and produce toxin in cooked food. Cornflour sauce in Norway and rice fried from boiled rice stock have been notable food vehicles.

The incubation period varies from 2 to 15 hours and the onset is sudden with acute vomiting and some diarrhoea; the symptoms soon abate. Long, warm storage, allowing multiplication of the organism to large numbers, is the fault leading to food poisoning.

Other aerobic spore bearers are described as agents of food poisoning, mostly in eastern Europe.

Escherichia coli

Escherichia coli is a normal inhabitant of the intestinal flora of man and animals. Certain serotypes are enteropathogenic and are known to cause diarrhoea in infants. Ingested in foods contaminated with large numbers, it is thought that particular strains cause diarrhoea in adults also. They will enter kitchens in many raw foodstuffs and readily pass to cooked foods by the usual means of hands, surfaces and containers and other equipment.

The incubation period is 1 to 3 days and the symptoms may resemble those of salmonella food poisoning or dysentery, when there is prolonged diarrhoea and blood and mucus in the stool.

There are other atypical coliform bacilli, including those of the Arizona group, which have been proved to cause food poisoning with symptoms similar to those given by organisms of the salmonella group.

Vibrio parahaemolyticus

In Japan an organism formerly designated *Pseudomonas*, *Oceanomonas* and even *Pasteurella* but now *Vibrio parahaemolyticus* is reported to cause 50 per cent or more of food poisoning incidents. In the warmer weather it can be isolated from fish, shell-fish and other seafoods and from coastal waters.

Reports of outbreaks have come from other countries also, including Korea, Vietnam, Australia, the United States and the United Kingdom. The organism has been isolated also from sea creatures and coastal waters of various countries, including the United Kingdom. Both raw and cooked foods, for example crab, have been vehicles of infection and it is suspected that cooked foods are contaminated by raw products.

The organism causes infection and the symptoms have been likened to those of both cholera and dysentery. The average incubation period is about 15 hours, and there is rapid onset of illness with profuse diarrhoea often leading to dehydration, vomiting and fever. The duration of illness is usually 2 to 5 days, although the ill-effects may linger on.

Other organisms

In addition to the seven groups of food poisoning organisms already described, other bacteria are sometimes reported as causal agents of food poisoning. Certain streptococci growing in foods in large numbers may produce toxins causing symptoms resembling but less acute than those from staphylococcal enterotoxin. *Proteus*, *Providencia* and *Pseudomonas* have all been implicated from time to time. Usually these organisms are isolated from suspected foods but not always from the faeces of patients, so that the evidence for their role in food poisoning is scanty, although serological tests may be used to support the diagnosis.

It seems that certain viruses are causing outbreaks of intestinal illness of a particular pattern but the investigation of faeces from such incidents has so far given inconclusive results except that other organisms known to cause food poisoning have not been found. The investigation of foodstuffs for viruses is carried out in some countries. Viruses cannot multiply in foods, only in certain living tissues; thus if viruses are agents of food poisoning their spread from the hands of human carriers and from water to foodstuffs is important, their incidence in foods grown in sewage-polluted water such as shell-fish and watercress may be relevant. There is little information about shared enteroviruses between animals and humans.

Some naturally occurring fungi are poisonous and the infestation of ground-nuts and other cereals by *Aspergillus flavus* can give rise to aflatoxin. Natural disease in turkey poults, ducklings, cattle, pigs, sheep and trout, and induced disease in laboratory animals have given rise to hepatic changes associated with liver carcinoma. Evidence that aflatoxin causes illness in man is scanty but there are a few reports of both acute and chronic illness. Information on toxic products, other than aflatoxin, from moulds is slowly becoming available but not many laboratories examine foods for these

TABLE 3. Presumed causes of food poisoning in 1969 and 1970 (England and Wales)

Presumed cause	1969 Number (%)		1970 Number (%)	
	Incidents	Cases*	Incidents	Cases†
Salmonella				
S. typhimurium	1,515‡ (31·0)	2,153 (23·2)	1,865 (35·3)	2,396 (27·7)
Other salmonellae§	3,305‡ (67·7)	5,169 (55·9)	3,360 (63·6)	4,456 (51·6)
Staphylococcus	17 (0·3)	397 (4·3)	29 (0·5)	523 (6·1)
Clostridium welchii	47 (1·0)	1,534 (16·6)	32 (0·6)	1,263 (14·6)
All agents	4,884‡	9,253	5,286	8,638

(Public Health Laboratory Service figures)

* Includes 261 symptomless excreters of S. *typhimurium* and 785 symptomless excreters of other salmonellae.
† Includes 361 symptomless excreters of S. *typhimurium* and 880 symptomless excreters of other salmonellae.
‡ Includes 3 outbreaks of mixed infection with S. *typhimurium* and other serotypes.
§ Excluding S. *typhi* and S. *paratyphi B.*

TABLE 4. Food poisoning in 1969 and 1970: Outbreaks, family outbreaks and sporadic cases by presumed causes
(England and Wales)

Presumed cause	Outbreaks		Family outbreaks		Sporadic cases		Total	
	1969	1970	1969	1970	1969	1970	1969	1970
Salmonella	139	138	607	636	4,074	4,451	4,820	5,225
Staphylococcus	14	18	3	4	0	7	17	29
Clostridium welchii	39	31	5	1	3	0	47	32
Total	192	187	615	641	4,077	4,458	4,884	5,286

(Public Health Laboratory Service figures)

substances. It seems that more attention should be given to the dangers of eating mouldy foods, whether contaminated through bad practice or intentionally. Fungi regularly employed for industrial purposes and in food manufacture should be carefully examined for toxic by-products. A Bibliography drawn up by the Tropical Products Institute in August 1964 (and later supplements) summa-rizes the literature on aflatoxin and other toxic products from fungi.

Table 3 gives the number of incidents and cases of food poisoning due to known bacterial agents notified in England and Wales for the years 1969 and 1970. Table 4 gives the distribution of causal agents of general outbreaks, family outbreaks and sporadic cases all due to known causes and notified in England and Wales for the years 1969 and 1970. An 'Outbreak' involves two or more related cases in persons of different families; a 'Family outbreak' involves two or more related cases in persons of the same family; and a 'Sporadic case' refers to a single case unrelated to any other.

It will be seen that, of all the incidents recorded, salmonellae and particularly *Salmonella typhimurium* were responsible for the majority, although sporadic cases accounted for a large number of the incidents due to salmonellae.

When the cause was definitely known the highest percentage of general outbreaks was due to salmonellae and *Cl. welchii*.

The total number of incidents (outbreaks and sporadic cases) reported in 1969 was 4,884 and the higher figure of 5,286 was recorded in 1970. The number of salmonella incidents due to *S. typhimurium* and other serotypes was higher in 1970 than 1969. It is interesting to note that the ratio between numbers of incidents due to *S. typhimurium* and other serotypes has changed since 1968; whereas *S. typhimurium* was predominant now the incidence of other serotypes has risen above that for *S. typhimurium*. Seventeen incidents of staphylococcal food poisoning occurred in 1969 compared with 29 in 1970 and the number of cases also increased. The number of recorded incidents due to *Cl. welchii* was 47 in 1969 and 32 in 1970. Outbreaks are reported mainly from canteens, hospitals, schools and other institutions where large numbers of persons may be affected. The ratio of the numbers of salmonella and *Cl. welchii* cases is closer than that of the numbers of incidents (Table 3) because of the larger proportion of sporadic cases of salmonellosis, each case of which is recorded as an incident.

It will be convenient now to consider in some detail the reservoirs of infection and the ways by which harmful bacteria are spread.

4
Reservoirs of Infection and Ways of Spread

Bacteria are everywhere in the environment, in soil, water, dust and air. Most of them are harmless but many can infect man and animals. Under certain conditions they are able to grow and multiply in the tissues of the body; some germs infect one tissue and some another. During illness it is well known that the infecting germs can be transferred from one person to another, from animal to animal, and from animal to man or man to animal, either directly or through a medium such as food. The fresh host may succumb to the disease, or he may resist it and show no symptoms although the infecting germ is harboured within his body for a variable period of time. In this way germs which are adapted to live under the conditions provided by the human or animal body maintain their existence and, when they are not actively causing disease, they may be surviving quietly in the nose, throat, or bowel of a healthy person or other living creature.

Some food poisoning is caused by the toxic products of bacteria growing actively in food and not by invasion of the body by the organism, for example staphylococcal food poisoning and botulism.

When it was first realized early in the twentieth century that bacteria were capable of causing food poisoning or food-borne disease, it was recognized that animals were the natural reservoirs of the salmonella group of intestinal organisms responsible for the majority of food-poisoning cases. The original investigations led workers to diseased animals as the source of contaminated meat (eaten by those affected), but subsequent workers have shown that the human and animal body may harbour organisms of the salmonella group without showing signs of disease. Also the human nose, throat and skin lesion are the main sources of staphylococci.

Foodstuffs of animal origin may be regarded as primary sources of food-poisoning bacteria; contamination passes from the live animal to the food during production either at home or abroad. The contaminated food as received is as much a hazard in food preparation areas as the living carrier.

31

The human and animal reservoir

Tables 5, 6 and 7 show the reservoirs and likely paths of spread from man and animals to food for the three main groups of food-poisoning organisms which frequently reside in living creatures.

The human nose, hand and skin

The primary habitat or natural home of staphylococci are the mucous membranes of the nose and the skin of man and animals. The left-hand side of Table 5 indicates the manner of spread of staphylococci from the human reservoir to food. We know that 30 to 50 per cent of non-institutional people carry staphylococci in the nose; in patients and working personnel in hospitals the nasal carriage may be as high as 60 to 80 per cent. Staphylococci may be isolated from the hands of 14 to 44 per cent of persons. There are many different types of staphylococci but they do not all produce the toxins responsible for food poisoning. Many of us touch the nose and mouth almost unconsciously, and from time to time handkerchiefs are used by everyone; nasal secretions are laden with bacteria, some of which may be staphylococci, and they are likely to contaminate the hands. Sometimes they penetrate into the deeper layers of the skin, where they may live and multiply in the pores and hair follicles. Hands so infected may be washed and scrubbed and yet continue to harbour staphylococci. In the hot, steamy atmosphere of the kitchen the pores are open and the organisms rise to the surface of the skin in the perspiration. We can try to rid the hands of staphylococci by using antiseptic lotions, hand creams or soaps, but there is no certain method of success although the number of organisms may be much reduced. There are preparations which are helpful in the treatment of the nasal carrier. It is better for food handlers who harbour staphylococci in the skin of their hands to avoid working with foodstuffs (such as cooked meats, milk and egg dishes) which encourage bacterial growth.

The pus from staphylococcal skin infections such as boils, carbuncles, whitlows, sycosis barbae (barber's rash) as well as septic cuts and burns will contain innumerable organisms, and a small speck of pus could inoculate food with millions of staphylococci.

Staphylococci like to live in cut surfaces; they thrive in the moist conditions provided by the serous fluid which is always present. Therefore the tiniest cut or abrasion, however clean and healthy it

TABLE 5. Human reservoirs of food-poisoning organisms

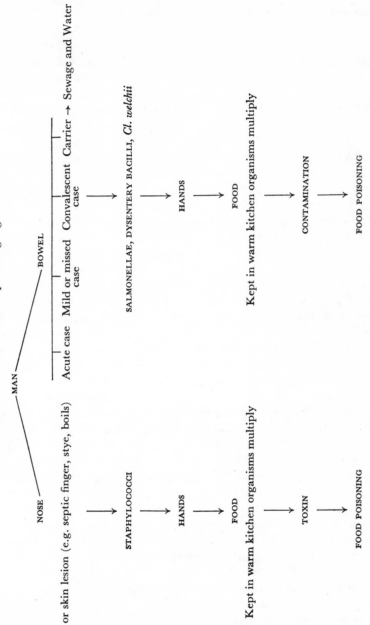

appears to be, may harbour many food-poisoning organisms and form a focus of infection.

There are many examples of outbreaks of staphylococcal food poisoning caused by the contamination of foods by staphylococci introduced from boils, ulcers, abrasions on the hands, and also from healthy looking hands. An infected trifle which caused acute illness among patients in a particular hospital ward was made by a chef with a varicose ulcer of the leg. The staphylococci growing profusely in the trifle were found to be of the same type as those infecting the ulcer.

The human and animal intestine

The right-hand side of Table 5 shows the chain of spread of salmonellae from the human reservoir. In any outbreak of infectious disease those who acquire the infection will react in one of four ways: a proportion will succumb to an acute illness; ambulant cases will exhibit symptoms so mild that they may be ignored or attributed to other indispositions; convalescent carriers will continue to excrete the organism after recovery from illness; temporary carriers or symptomless excreters may harbour the infecting germ for a short time without exhibiting symptoms.

Aerosol sprays from flushed lavatory pans, soiled seats, pull chains, door handles and taps may pass infection from person to person. The more fluid the stool the more danger from spread. Contaminated hands may pass infection to food. These intestinal organisms are readily washed from the hands by soap and water. They are not harboured in the skin like staphylococci.

Hands will also transmit bacteria from food to food. Fig. 8 shows finger print cultures of colonies of bacteria from unwashed and washed hands and from hands after holding a moist scouring sponge and after touching raw chicken. It will be noted that there are moderate numbers of bacteria on a dry hand before washing but that many and various bacteria are picked up from a moist kitchen sponge and raw chicken and that immediately after washing the hand is by no means sterile.

It is often asked how long after infection people remain carriers and continue to excrete infective organisms; this will depend on the type of organism. The excretion of *Salmonella typhi* may persist for many years, while other salmonella serotypes and dysentery bacilli are excreted for a few weeks only, rarely months and only exceptionally for a year or more. Treatment of persistent excreters

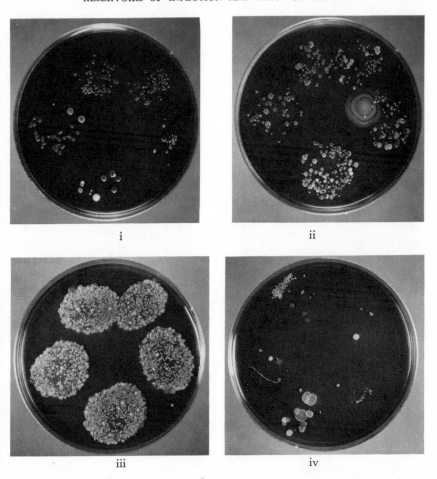

FIG. 8. Colonies of bacteria from finger prints of washed and unwashed hands.
   i. Dry hand before washing
  ii. Hand after touching moist scouring sponge
 iii. Hand after touching raw chicken
 iv. Hand immediately after washing

with antibiotics is not recommended because it tends to prolong the excretion and encourage resistance of the organisms.

The sources of *Clostridium welchii* are likely to be both human and animal in a cycle similar to that shown in Table 6; 'animal' includes poultry and 'meat' includes poultry meat.

Table 7 gives the names of the animals known to be occasional or persistent reservoirs of organisms of the salmonella group. Animals may suffer from salmonella infections or become transient symptomless excreters in the same way as human beings. They may become infected through eating contaminated feeding meals, grazing on contaminated pasture land or by contact with animal, human or bird excreters on the farm, during transport or in the lairage of markets or slaughterhouses. It has been observed that a far higher proportion of pigs and sheep, for example, excrete salmonellae when under conditions of stress, excitement, fear or privation, than

TABLE 6. Human and animal reservoirs of *Clostridium welchii*

ANIMAL   HUMAN

FLY

EXCRETA

FLY,
SOIL, DUST

CARCASS   HANDS

RAW MEAT

Spores survive cooking,
germinate and multiply during
cooling and storage

GROSSLY CONTAMINATED MEAT

FOOD POISONING

during normal day-to-day life on the farm. As well as animal-to-animal spread of infected excreta there may be direct soiling of food such as from cow to milk and meat, pig to meat, from poultry to the shells of eggs and from vermin and domestic pets to all kinds of food.

Organisms from infected carcasses may be transferred to other meat in the slaughterhouse, during transport and in the butcher's shop or manufacturing establishment. A widespread outbreak of salmonella food poisoning in 1947 illustrates the danger of cross-contamination from one meat to another. There were about 3,000 to 4,000 cases with 3 deaths and the origin of infection was thought to be one infected pig or it may well have been a number of infected

TABLE 7. Animal reservoirs of salmonella organisms

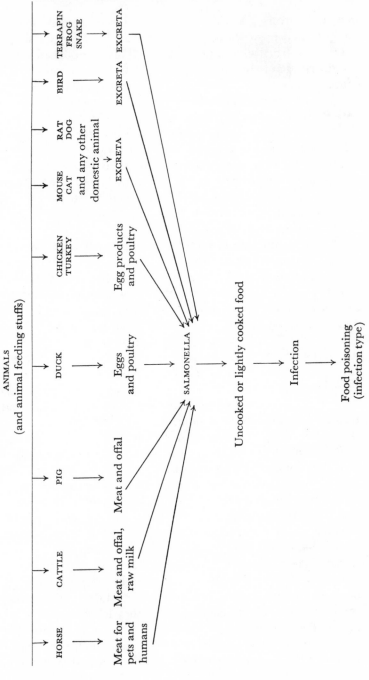

pigs, the carcasses of which contaminated other carcasses in the slaughterhouse by various means, particularly by the spreading of infection from wiping-down cloths. This home-killed raw meat was distributed to butchers' shops and handled in conjunction with canned meat. The infected raw meat and the cold meats were weighed on the same balance, cut with the same knife and handled with the same hands; there was, therefore, plenty of opportunity for the spread of infection. The contamination of the pressed beef and other cooked meats was responsible for the widespread nature of the outbreak, for these meats were eaten without further heat treatment—often after storage at a temperature favourable for bacterial multiplication. In 1960 home-killed infected veal used for manufactured products and retail sale caused a number of cases of salmonellosis in England.

The contamination rate of carcass meat will vary according to the proportion of animals excreting salmonellae and the hygiene of the meat establishment. There has been an increase in the number of calves and cattle infected with S. typhimurium, associated with the mass production of animals on farms using intensive rearing methods. Many strains are resistant to antibiotics which may be used liberally in feeds for prophylactic reasons to stem the intestinal infections which afflict intensively-kept calves. It has now been shown that drug resistance may be passed from cell to cell and from one species of organism to another so that there is an ever-increasing danger of the spread of antibiotic-resistant salmonellae and the transfer of resistance to organisms producing other human infections. The British Medical Journal suggested a revision in farming practice and the use of drugs. In 1969 the Joint Committee on the use of Antibiotics in Animal Husbandry and Veterinary Medicine made the following recommendations: 'antibiotics used for treatment of humans should not be used in feeds for animals nor for prophylaxis'.

Horses have been shown to excrete salmonellae, and frozen boneless horsemeat imported for pet food can be a major source of salmonellae. Salmonellae have been found also in a high proportion of samples of imported frozen boneless kangaroo meat. Without careful handling and cooking of the meats the organism is likely to spread in domestic kitchens so that other foods may be contaminated. Pets themselves as excreters may infect children playing with them; furthermore, the fly population alighting on infected excreta may carry the germs back into the house. In many countries

TABLE 8. Salmonella in raw meat (1961–1965)

Raw meat and offal	Number of samples examined	Positive for salmonellae	
		Number	Per cent
Wholesale (imported)			
Frozen boneless			
veal	1,328	192	14·4
beef	3,420	410	11·9
beef offal	102	9	8·8
mutton	1,107	123	11·1
mutton offal	155	4	2·5
horse	12,406	4,516	36·4
horse offal	1,031	421	40·8
kangaroo	929	410	44·1
Retail (English and imported)			
butcher's shop meat	262	4	1·5
butcher's shop offal	52	0	—
pet shop meat	433	120	27·7
pet shop offal	148	25	16·9
knacker's yard meat	64	7	10·9

horse meat is eaten by the human population; in the United Kingdom, although mainly sold for pets, it is sometimes seen raw alongside meat and fish in retail shops, and may be dispensed with the same equipment as that used for fish or other meats. Meat from knackers' yards, condemned for human consumption but sold raw for pets, has been the source of salmonellae causing outbreaks of salmonellosis amongst families owning pets. In 1969 a new law was passed, The Meat (Sterilization) Regulations, 1969, to ensure that condemned meat, whether imported or home produced, intended for animals, be cooked before sale. Canned pet foods, sterilized by heat treatment during the canning process, should be safe. Table 8 gives results for the salmonella contamination of various meats.

Poultry are known to be major reservoirs of salmonella organisms and the shell of hens' eggs may be contaminated through contact with the faeces in the cloaca or in the nest or battery. The organisms may penetrate the shell under certain conditions of humidity and temperature. Though this may be an uncommon occurrence, one infected egg may contaminate batches of liquid egg broken out in bulk for freezing or drying. Also fragments of shell or specks of dirt may fall into the mixture; the hands of those breaking out will contaminate the equipment and the mix. Even when liquid egg is dried, organisms remain viable since the temperatures reached are not high enough or sustained for long enough to kill them. Methods of treatment to render these products free from infection will be described in Chapter 5.

The salmonella contamination of spray-dried whole egg was first discovered during the war years of 1939 to 1945 when outbreaks of salmonellosis were traced to this source. The presence of the same types of salmonellae in the faeces, mesenteric glands and flesh of pigs was shown to be due to the consumption of dried whole egg by pigs. Some years later outbreaks of enteric fever and salmonellosis due to salmonellae including paratyphoid bacilli were traced to the use of Chinese frozen whole egg for cakes in bakeries preparing imitation cream cakes also (see Chapter 5). It was soon discovered that a proportion of all egg products, whole, white or yolk, broken out in bulk for the liquid, frozen or dried materials were contaminated with salmonellae.

Although salmonellae are not commonly found in the yolk or white of hens' eggs in shell, the yolk of ducks' eggs is not infrequently infected. It seems that in the duck the oviduct, where the egg is formed, may become infected. The duck is a notorious scavenger and it is possible that in the course of the day's activities, which include swimming in a pond which may be contaminated by other birds or rats, the infected material is picked up, ingested, and transferred from the digestive tract to the oviduct. The drake may spread the infection from bird to bird.

Unlike the hen, which likes to keep dry, the duck frequently lays eggs in wet and muddy places, so that the shell may be particularly susceptible to penetration by bacteria. Whatever the cause, it is known that ducks' eggs are fairly frequently contaminated. They should, therefore, be used with caution and regarded as a possible source of danger even though they look and smell normal. The recommendations given for the use of ducks' eggs in cooking (see Chapter 11) should be strictly carried out.

Poultry as well as other farm animals, such as cattle and pigs, are exposed to infection from feeding meals; many of these are known to contain salmonellae which may lead to a transient carrier state or sometimes to actual disease. The rapid growth of the broiler industry for chickens, turkeys and ducks seems to be associated with increased infection of birds and carcasses. There is likely to be a higher proportion of poultry carcasses contaminated during bulk handling than by small-scale operations. The spread of contamination may be aggravated by modern methods of retail cooking, storage and packaging.

Milk-borne infection has been largely eliminated by pasteurization, but outbreaks of food poisoning due to salmonellae and staphylococcal enterotoxin still occur from raw TT milk infected by cows or humans.

Desiccated coconut is another food that may be contaminated by salmonellae of human or animal origin during various stages in production; when used to garnish it can be responsible for introducing salmonellae, including paratyphoid bacilli. Improved methods of production have considerably reduced if not eliminated the hazard.

Vermin and birds

Rats and mice can suffer from infection due to types of salmonellae which infect man, and they can also become symptomless excreters; in either case their excreta are a source of danger to food which they soil. It is known that a proportion of the vermin population become intestinal carriers of salmonellae, in the same way as described for other animals and for man. The organisms will be picked up on farms, in sewers and from garbage.

In the past certain vermin poisons were lethal because they contained virulent organisms of the salmonella group. The danger from the use of such material is obvious and in fact outbreaks occurred in various parts of the world owing to accidental contamination of human food with the 'poisons'; furthermore, a proportion of the animals it was intended to kill undoubtedly survived and became excreters. In Britain the sale of this material is forbidden; there are many poisons more effective for animals and harmless to human beings (Chapter 15).

Wild birds excrete salmonellae in proportion to the foods eaten by them. The scavenger type, for example sea gulls and even pigeons feeding on urban waste from tips and sewage outflows, are frequently infected; whereas salmonellae are rarely found in country birds in sparsely populated areas.

Domestic animals

In Britain approximately 1 to 2 per cent of cats and dogs were found to be excreting salmonellae without symptoms in 1956; the proportion may be far higher now because of the increased practice of feeding raw horsemeat, which is known to be a source of salmonellae, to domestic pets; in the USA 15 per cent of dogs fed meat and bone meal (rarely free from salmonellae) were found to be excreters. These results suggest that Food Hygiene Regulations which ban the presence of cats and dogs in retail food shops are justified.

The widespread distribution to farm animals of contaminated feeding meals may lead to transitory infection of a proportion of animals over a large area. In some circumstances when animal husbandry is good no harm may be done, but in particular instances there may be spread of infection in herds combined with poor hygiene in slaughterhouses. Contaminated carcasses may lead to contaminated manufactured products, and particularly raw comminuted meats such as sausages.

The sources of infection on farms are likely to be threefold:

1. animal excreters as foci of infection;
2. feeding stuffs;
3. environmental factors including man, other animals, vermin, birds and water.

It may be assumed that if the feeding stuffs were rendered safe, the importance of (1) and (3) would be reduced also. The movement of animals such as calves for breeding purposes and pigs for mating may be a big factor in the spread of infection under present conditions.

In a survey of cattle, 21 per cent of 4,496 swabs from abattoir drains were positive for salmonellae; isolations were most frequent where a high proportion of cattle were slaughtered.

The same salmonella serotypes and even the same phage types of *S. typhimurium* were found in abattoirs and also in human cases of salmonellosis in the areas served by the abattoirs. These findings indicated that contaminated meat products were sold in the local shops. In 8 food poisoning incidents, 281 cases and excreters, there was convincing evidence that meat or a meat product was the vehicle of infection. In a further 23 incidents meat-borne infection was likely. Cattle and pigs were important foci of infection and the meat from pigs, cattle and calves was a source of infection and responsible for both sporadic cases and outbreaks of disease.

Salmonellae were isolated from 2 to 14 per cent of 5,637 pigs in the southwest of England. The majority of serotypes were similar to those found in feeding stuffs and those causing food poisoning in the human population, such as *S. typhimurium, S. dublin, S. panama, S. livingstone, S. stanley, S. fischerkietz, S. bredeney, S. indiana, S. heidelberg, S. anatum, S. senftenberg,* and *S. montevideo.*

A comparative study made in Denmark, where there is legislation compelling treatment to free feeding stuffs from salmonellae, showed that the incidence of salmonellae in pigs was lower than in England and the majority of serotypes common in pigs in England were not found, nor were they found in the human population in Denmark.

Other ways in which infection spreads to food

Flies have always been considered as a major factor in the spread of infection; no doubt they still play a part, but in countries where they are, for the most part, controlled and sanitation is good, the direct contamination of foods by human beings and animals is more important.

Where sanitation is poor and intestinal diseases such as dysentery, typhoid and paratyphoid fever are endemic, an abundance of flies is a far greater menace. There is ready access to infected excreta from cases and carriers, and they can transfer disease-producing bacteria to foodstuffs.

In western countries where sanitation is good there are still untidy dustbins with ill-fitting lids or no lids at all in the back premises of private houses, blocks of flats, restaurants, hotels, canteens and other premises which prepare foodstuffs; often they are placed outside kitchen windows.

The fly can feed on unwrapped waste and regurgitate its meals on to foodstuffs in the kitchen; it may also carry particles of infected material on its feet, from the waste-bin to foods. The house-fly and the stable-fly, as well as the larger type of bluebottle and greenbottle, may transfer infection in this way. *Clostridium welchii* has been isolated from many batches of greenbottle and bluebottle flies.

There are other insects, particularly the cockroach, which can also carry food-poisoning bacteria from place to place. An Australian article describes an outbreak of salmonellosis amongst children in a hospital where flies, cockroaches and mice were all found to be carrying the organism responsible for the infection. It was not suggested that these creatures were the original source but that they had picked up the bacteria from the contaminated environment. It was thought that contaminated wash water from ward sinks used for washing hands and infant clothing was splashed on to the surrounding floor and pipes. Cockroaches walking over these areas would pick up bacteria and convey them from place to place on their feet and bodies.

In general, however, cockroaches are less likely to harbour infection than flies because they breed in wall cracks and paper rather than refuse and manure heaps. Likewise, wasps, bees, spiders and similar creatures, because of their different breeding grounds, are unlikely to carry harmful bacteria and, compared with flies, their habits are less unhygienic.

Inanimate objects such as towels, pencils, door handles, WC equipment, crockery and cutlery may serve as intermediate objects in the transfer of infection from person to person, or from person to food. Roller towels may be dangerous; if the hands are not washed thoroughly, dirt containing bacteria will be left on the towel to be picked up by the next person to use it. The discharge from staphylococcal infections (for example boils, barber's rash and other septic spots present on the face, hands or arms of canteen personnel) may be left on communal towels. The spread of boils throughout a factory has been encouraged in this way. It has sometimes been suggested that a towel or other object shared by people was responsible for the passage of salmonellae from a carrier or food to a food handler.

Door handles, pull grips on chains and other WC equipment should be constructed of material which will not permit the survival of bacteria; most metals are self-sterilizing, and they should be used in preference to wood, rubber or plastic.

Where practicable a pedal-operated water supply both for hand washing and for flushing toilets should be installed for hygienic reasons.

Money is frequently thought to spread infection. Coins of copper, silver or nickel are commonly self-sterilizing but banknotes, newspapers and other used paper may harbour living bacteria. Care should be taken not to lick the fingers and so apply saliva and mouth organisms before picking up paper money or paper for wrapping food.

Bacteria from crockery, cutlery and cloths may be transferred to those using them or to foodstuffs, although it is almost impossible to trace outbreaks of infection which have originated or spread in this manner. Recommended methods for washing crockery and cutlery will be given in Chapter 12.

5

The Vehicle of Infection

The bacteria responsible for food-borne infection or food poisoning may be transferred from animal hosts to foodstuffs where they may grow and multiply. The resistant spores of bacteria and moulds survive indefinitely in dust and soil and so they are present on and within many foods. Some foods, both solid and liquid, are readily contaminated and favourable for the growth of bacteria, while others are not.

Each year the same categories of food figure prominently in the statistics for bacterial food poisoning; these foods encourage the growth of bacteria whereas highly salted, sugary and acid foods do not cause food poisoning because they are unsatisfactory media for growth.

The dose of bacteria necessary to infect or to produce sufficient toxin to cause symptoms varies with different organisms and also with the resistance of the person who swallows the food. The number of organisms in a particular food substance at any given time will depend on the nature of the foodstuff, its temperature and the length of time it has been kept.

There are a small number of poisoning incidents each year from chemicals. Nicotine and ascorbic acid added to raw minced meat to maintain an appearance of freshness, zinc from galvanized iron or corroded containers, copper from worn tinned containers, antimony from chipped enamel, tin from old cans of fruit are reported occasionally in poisoning incidents. There are rare accidents from pesticides and other materials used in agriculture.

Meat and poultry

Since records for food poisoning have been kept, meat and poultry have been proved to be the food vehicles responsible for most outbreaks. In 80 to 90 per cent of incidents for which a cause was established, a meat or poultry dish is incriminated. Table 9 summarizes the food vehicle of infection of 88 general and family outbreaks in 1969 and 91 outbreaks in 1970 in England and Wales, and Table 10 classifies the meat and poultry products according to their treatment in processing and cooking.

TABLE 9. Vehicles of food-poisoning infection (England and Wales) 1969 and 1970

Vehicle	Incidents			
	1969		1970	
	Number	Per cent	Number	Per cent
Meat and poultry	77	87·5	75	82·4 (see Table 10)
Sweet	2	2·3 (*Staphylococcus*)	2	2·2 (*Staphylococcus*)
Milk unpasteurized	4	4·6 (*Salmonella*)	10	11·0 (*Salmonella*)
Cream pasteurized	1	1·1 (*Salmonella*)	0	
Sea food frozen prawns	1	1·1 (*Staphylococcus*)	1	1·1 (*Staphylococcus*)
Vegetable pease pudding / creamed potatoes / canned peas	0 / 1 / 1 } 2	2·3 (*Staphylococcus*)	2 / 0 / 0 } 2	2·2 (*Cl. welchii*)
Egg duck	1	1·1 (*Salmonella*)	0	
Sauce butter	0		1	1·1 (*Staphylococcus*)
Total	88		91	

TABLE 10. Food poisoning 1970: General and family outbreaks associated with processed or made-up meats

	Presumed causal agents			
Vehicle of infection	Salmon-ella	Staphy-lococcus	Cl. welchii	All agents
Reheated meat				
Poultry	3	1	2	6
Stew, including mince	—	—	6	6
Beef	—	—	4	4
Pork	1	—	1	2
Mutton	—	1	2	3
Cold meat				
Processed meat:				
Ham, boiled bacon	2	9	—	11
Tongue	—	1	—	1
Fresh meat:				
Poultry	9	5	2	16
Beef	2	—	3	5
Pork	4	—	—	4
Cooked meats	1	—	1	2
Roast meat, not stated to have been reheated or served cold				
Poultry	5	—	2	7
Mutton	—	—	1	1
Meat pies				
Manufactured:				
Pasties	—	1	—	1
Other	1	—	—	1
Made at home or canteen:				
Shepherd's pie	—	—	2	2
Vol-au-vent	—	—	2	2
Steak	—	—	1	1
Total	28	18	29	75

(Public Health Laboratory Service figures)

It is clear that if freshly cooked, roasted, boiled or fried meats and poultry exclusively were eaten hot, sporadic cases and outbreaks of food poisoning would be considerably reduced. The preparation of meat products for eating and the periods of storage between preparation and eating contributes to the contamination leading to food poisoning. In the Tables preparative treatment includes curing and is referred to as 'processed and made up'; Table 10 shows that the bulk of the incidents fall into this group.

In the analysis of general and family outbreaks according to food and causal agents given in Table 10, the reheated foods are predominant vehicles followed by the cold meats and poultry. The reheated meats are usually fresh meats which have been cooked some time before required and eaten warmed up or cold. In the reheated group, except for salmonella food poisoning from poultry, *Clostridium welchii* is the common causal agent. The survival of the spores through cooking and subsequent outgrowth and multiplication is encouraged by storage and warming up procedures. The same applies to home- and canteen-made pies and pasties when the meat is precooked.

The cold meats are subdivided into cured and uncured meats. Both are subject to much handling and thus to contamination with staphylococci from the hands. Staphylococcal outbreaks occur mainly from cold cooked meats, including the manufactured-cured products because staphylococci grow readily in meats with an abnormal salt content from curing solutions. The organisms usually come from food handlers involved in production or responsible for slicing and service. There are many different kinds of cold cooked meats and there is ample opportunity for contamination either during preparation or while the meats are stored in the retail shop or consumer's kitchen. Contamination may take place during manufacture, in the shop or kitchen from hands, utensils, slicing machines and scales, and subsequent storage may encourage multiplication. Most of these products are eaten cold or merely warmed up.

The sources of the majority of salmonella serotypes which reach foods is the raw product. Poultry and comminuted meats are frequently contaminated with salmonellae as they enter the kitchen and it is not difficult to imagine the spread of infection from raw to cooked products via hands, surfaces, equipment such as chopping blocks, cutting boards and slicing machines, various

TABLE 11. Major outbreaks of *Clostridium welchii* and staphylococcal food poisoning from meat dishes (England and Wales) 1967–1970

Year	Place	Type of meat	Infective organisms	Number of persons affected
1967	Islington	Reheated roast lamb	*Cl. welchii*	35
	Lichfield	Cold brisket of beef	*Cl. welchii*	108
	Lichfield	Cold brisket of beef	*Cl. welchii*	120
	Wandsworth	Cold chicken vol-au-vent	*Cl. welchii*	67
	Devizes	Cold boiled tongue	*Cl. welchii*	68
	Bethesda	Cold boiled ox tongue	Staphylococcal	31
	Llandudno	Cold boiled ham	Staphylococcal	61
	Wallasey	Reheated roast lamb	*Cl. welchii*	30
	Stockton	Boiled brisket of beef	*Cl. welchii*	100
	Winchester	Reheated mince	*Cl. welchii*	60
	Worsley	Cold boiled tongue	*Cl. welchii*	26
1968	Stretford	Reheated hotpot	*Cl. welchii*	30
	Manchester	Reheated roast turkey	*Cl. welchii*	87
	Bredbury & Romilly	Ox heart and stock	*Cl. welchii*	30
	Richmond-on Thames	Cold boiled beef	*Cl. welchii*	25
	Hemsworth	Boiled minced kidney	*Cl. welchii*	200
	Bridgwater	Steak and kidney pudding	*Cl. welchii*	24
	Sheffield	Reheated beef in gravy	*Cl. welchii*	42
	Cheltenham	Corned beef	*Cl. welchii*	111
	Southampton	Steak pie	*Cl. welchii*	43
	Bedwellty	Cold roast beef	*Cl. welchii*	63
	Hazel Grove	Reheated roast lamb	*Cl. welchii*	158
	Bury	Cold roast beef	*Cl. welchii*	21
	Whitefield	Reheated steam-roasted chicken	*Cl. welchii*	85
1969	Worsley	Reheated roast lamb	*Cl. welchii*	23
	Pontypool	Cold roast beef	*Cl. welchii*	63
	Chichester	Reheated chicken vol-au-vent	Staphylococcal	25
	Bradford	Cold chicken and ham	Staphylococcal	63
	Hammersmith	Chicken and ham vol-au-vent	Staphylococcal	50
	Norman Cross	Cold roast chicken	Staphylococcal	30
	Hastings	Reheated roast pork	*Cl. welchii*	50
	Worthing and Kensington	Cold beef, tongue and ham	Staphylococcal	38
	Colwyn Bay	Cold brisket of beef	*Cl. welchii*	26
	Alton	Reheated roast turkey	*Cl. welchii*	20

TABLE 11—*continued*

Year	Place	Type of meat	Infective organisms	Number of persons affected
1970	Bletchley	Cold tongue	Staphylococcal	141
	Axbridge	Ham	Staphylococcal	35
	Hackney	Cold boiled ham	Staphylococcal	31
	Hove	Chicken	*Cl. welchii*	144
	Brighton	Ham in rolls	Staphylococcal	50
	Ponterdawe	Reheated mince	*Cl. welchii*	145
	Dartford	Reheated pease pudding	*Cl. welchii*	186
	Leigh	Cold turkey and ham	Staphylococcal	40
	Teesside	Cold boiled chicken	*Cl. welchii*	70
	Southampton	Turkey	*Cl. welchii*	70
	Aberbargoed	Cold boiled beef	*Cl. welchii*	48
	Abercarn	Cold boiled beef	*Cl. welchii*	61

utensils and cloths. Food handlers may be victims of the foods they are preparing for the table and become sources of infection.

Meals including fresh meat and poultry eaten cold or reheated and home- or canteen-produced pies have been predominant in causing *Cl. welchii* food poisoning. In large canteen kitchens meat frequently is cooked, allowed to cool slowly at atmospheric temperature and stored in a cool or cold room overnight. The following day it is served cold, warmed up, sliced in hot gravy, or made into pies, pasties, or meat puddings. This practice is dangerous for two reasons. In meats cooked at a temperature not higher than 100 °C (212 °F), for example, boiled, stewed, braised, steamed and lightly roasted meats, spores of *Cl. welchii* may survive cooking and, in slowly cooling meat, germinate into actively multiplying bacterial cells able to cause food poisoning. Because heat penetrates into meat very slowly, large cuts of meat (over 6 lb; 2·7 kg) are particularly dangerous. With rolled meat the outside may become contaminated and, when folded inside, may not be heated sufficiently to destroy the contaminating organism. Also, cooked meats and poultry carved cold may be contaminated during slicing or other manipulation carried out with the help of the fingers.

Table 11 gives some recent outbreaks caused by the growth in meats of staphylococci and *Cl. welchii*.

The contamination of raw meat, particularly boneless packed meat, with salmonellae has already been described in Chapter 4. The danger of cross-contamination by spread of infection from raw meats to cooked foods or to foods eaten without cooking is apparent.

The irradiation of frozen packs of boneless horsemeat with small doses of gamma-rays will successfully eliminate salmonellae. The method, as yet unsanctioned, might be considered for all packs of frozen boneless meats for human and animal consumption when the usual hygienic methods fail to prevent contamination.

Canned food

Canned food rarely causes food poisoning unless the contents of the can are contaminated with food-poisoning bacteria after the can has been opened. The general standard of canning is high and it is unusual to find that under-processed cans or cans with structural defects have reached the kitchen.

Occasionally, however, there are manufacturing faults leading to small leaks in the seams of cans, and the seams may be strained during the heat processing of the food. If unclean water is used to cool the cans after heat treatment organisms may be sucked through the holes, and if the food and conditions of storage are suitable, the bacteria will grow and cause spoilage or perhaps food poisoning. Bacteria (for example, staphylococci) from the hands may be sucked through leaks when wet cans are transported by hand from the retort to trolleys or storage places. Cans of food stored in a moist atmosphere may rust and develop holes through which organisms may pass at any time. Spoiled or blown cans, bulged at either or both ends, rarely reach the public because they are usually discovered by the manufacturer before leaving the factory or by health inspectors during routine visits to retail shops. Yet food-poisoning organisms may grow inside cans without gas production or any obvious signs of spoilage. Thus great care is needed both with the manufacture and sealing of cans and with the processing times and temperatures required for sterility. Outbreaks of typhoid fever in England and Scotland have been caused by canned meat contaminated with typhoid bacilli from polluted cooling water. Typhoid bacilli grow well and spread in canned corned beef and they can survive in the can for at least 8 years (see Chapters 6 and 8).

Products such as corned beef, stewed steak and vegetables are processed at pressures calculated to give temperatures well above boiling, and known to destroy most heat-resistant bacterial spores, such as those of *Cl. botulinum*, and these products should be sterile. Many canned meats including chopped pork, jellied veal, and tongue are not processed at such high temperatures because it is desired to preserve the maximum bulk and aesthetic qualities of appearance and palatability. The contents of these lightly treated cans may not be sterile and their shelf life is limited. A third category of canned meats includes the shoulders and hams of pork which are heated at 'pasteurization' temperatures only, to avoid shrinkage and loss of flavour. They are not sterile; but there is a recommendation that after the heat process there should not be more than 10,000 per g of heat-resistant spores present and all vegetative cells should be killed. Good manufacturers of canned meat will ensure the lowest possible bacterial population by care in production and the preparation of meat from freshly slaughtered animals, combined with well balanced pickling solutions to inhibit growth. The maximum time and temperatures should be given to eliminate all but heat-resistant sporing organisms, which are unlikely to develop in well-cured products. All non-sterile canned meats should be labelled 'Perishable, keep in a cold place'; it is important for these products to be stored cold. International recommendations for minimum standards of heat treatment, salt and nitrite content would be safeguards against hazards due to the careless use of this method of processing.

Foods for canning are usually of good quality and fresh; they are packed and sealed in airtight containers frequently lacquered to prevent interaction between the foodstuff and the tinplate, which may cause discoloration.

The belief that foodstuffs must not remain in opened tins arose from the fear of interaction between the foodstuff, meat container and air. Tinplate has much improved and the lacquer on the inside is an added protection. Foods may be safely stored in the opened can for a few days, particularly if refrigerated. It must be remembered, however, that foods from opened cans are susceptible to bacteria from any source and to contamination from persons handling them.

Sterilized packs of canned meat may be kept for 5 years; cans of veal and carrots in gravy, retrieved from one of Sir Edward Parry's expeditions in search of the Northwest Passage, were wholesome after 115 years. Some canned foods should not be stored as long as 5 years, because slow chemical changes may occur; for example, the limit for milk should be 1 year, vegetables 2 years; canned fish in oil withstands 5 years' storage, but the limit for fish in tomato sauce is 1 year. A regular yearly turnover for all canned foods is advisable; therefore the date of purchase should be written on the cans.

Cans should be stored in a cool, dry place, as high temperatures may alter flavour and colour, and dampness will cause rust and may lead to perforations; badly bashed cans may perforate also. Once opened, a can of meat should be kept covered and cold and the contents eaten soon. It must be remembered also that cans which show bulges at the ends are blown and should be discarded without hesitation.

Dairy products (milk, fresh cream, cheese and eggs)

Milk

A substantial portion of urban England and Wales is now covered by directions requiring the heat treatment of all milk other than that produced under conditions enabling it to be sold as 'Untreated' formerly Tuberculin Tested. In 1969 there were 4 and in 1970 10 outbreaks of food poisoning from salmonella organisms consumed in unpasteurized milk. In some episodes the same phage types of S. typhimurium have been isolated from calves, cows, milk and people; sometimes salmonellae were found in farm manure and water. Examples of outbreaks are given in Chapters 6 and 8.

The cow's udder is a common source of food-poisoning staphylococci which are found in most samples of raw milk and therefore in dairy products made with unheated or lightly heated milk. Nevertheless milk-borne outbreaks of staphylococcal food poisoning are not common; there may be one (1962) or two (1961) in a year confined to raw TT milk. Tests for detecting traces of antibiotics in milk are statutory in some countries and in England and Wales action may be taken under the Food and Drugs Act, where a concentration of penicillin greater than 0·05 i.u. per ml is not permitted.

Fresh cream

There are few outbreaks traced to fresh cream produced in the UK, although in the USA cream seems to be a common vehicle for staphylococcal food poisoning. Cream may be prepared from raw milk, from pasteurized milk, or it may be pasteurized after separation but before bottling. A minority of creameries carry out in-bottle pasteurization. Cream may be filled into bottles and cartons at the creamery or it may be transported in cans or churns for filling at distribution centres. A survey of the bacteriological condition of cream, sampled mostly from retail shops, indicated that there was a high degree of post-pasteurization contamination but the samples which had been heat treated again after pasteurization were almost sterile.

It has been suggested that the introduction of a grading scheme for cream similar to that for ice-cream and based on advisory tests for keeping quality would draw attention to unsuitable supplies so that methods of processing, storage in bulk, transportation and retail storage could be improved.

Cheese

A more serious problem may arise when cheese is prepared from raw or inadequately heated milk. Commercially prepared natural cheese is made by the acidification of milk using bacterial cultures, combined with clotting by rennet. The increasing veterinary use of antibiotics for treatment of disease, including staphylococcal mastitis in cows, has resulted firstly in traces of antibiotics remaining in the milk and secondly in the development of resistance to the antibiotics by the staphylococcus. Sometimes, for this and other reasons, the starter culture fails to grow whereas the staphylococci, frequently present in raw milk, survive and multiply freely. Outbreaks of staphylococcal food poisoning have occurred in factories and hospitals through eating cheese contaminated in this way. The cheese has usually been classified as second grade because of its abnormal flavour resulting from the failure of the starter culture to grow; such cheese is imported for blending and processing and is not intended for consumption without treatment.

The pasteurization of all milk, including the tuberculin tested class, whether intended for drinking or for the production of cream or cheese, greatly reduces the hazard of food poisoning from this source. In 1963 New Zealand introduced legislation to compel the pasteurization of milk for making cheese.

'Cream' cheeses have always constituted a risk when prepared from raw milk but most proprietary brands are prepared from heat-treated milk.

Eggs

The contamination of eggs by salmonellae has already been described in Chapter 4 and the results of examination of ducks' and hens' eggs (shell) are given in Tables 12 and 13. It may be seen that the isolation of salmonellae from both ducks' and hens' eggs is variable. The amount of infection in the parent poultry flock probably depends on the degree of contamination of the feeding stuffs and environmental factors. Nevertheless, the contamination of ducks' eggs with salmonellae is more consistent, as shown by the results of examination of melange from broken out eggs. Between 1951 and 1955 in Northern Ireland salmonellae were isolated from 48 per cent of batches of duck egg mix compared with 2 per cent of batches of hen egg mix; the batches usually contained between 4,000 and 20,000 eggs. Another group of workers in England found salmonellae in 2 of 65 samples of liquid duck egg and 6 of 1,649 samples of liquid hen egg. Later the contamination of hen egg products in bulk, such as liquid, frozen and dried whole, white and yolk, was found to be more common and salmonellae were found in the products of many countries. Results obtained in 1961 and 1962 are given in Table 14. By 1963 some countries were testing the practicability of pasteurization, and, of 829 samples from pasteurized whole egg from four countries, only 5 (0·6 per cent) showed salmonellae, whereas of 800 raw unpasteurized samples 136 (17 per cent) were positive for salmonellae.

TABLE 12. Salmonellae from ducks' eggs (shell). Historical record (excluding *S. pullorum* and *S. gallinarum*)

Year	Country	Number examined	Number positive	Serotype
1932	England	166	7	*S. enteritidis*
1934	Germany	1,500	15	Salmonellae
1936	Germany	332	19	*S. typhimurium*
1944	England	2,000	0	
1945	England	16	3	*S. typhimurium*
1950–52	England	13,562	20	*S. typhimurium* *S. enteritidis*
1951–63	All countries	?	10	*S. typhimurium*
1963	All countries	?	5	*S. thompson*

The large-scale investigation of imported and home-produced egg products revealed the fact that these contaminated ingredients were sources of infection in bakeries leading to widely distributed outbreaks of paratyphoid fever and salmonella food poisoning.

Outbreaks resulted from the accidental contamination of uncooked products such as imitation cream prepared in the same bowls and with the same utensils as the egg mixes used in the baked ingredients.

Bulked liquid egg is now made safe in England and Wales by compulsory pasteurization at 64·4°C (148°F) for 2½ minutes in a manner similar to that used for milk; the heat treatment does not adversely affect the baking properties of the egg. Destruction of the enzyme alpha-amylase in the yolk of the egg is used as a test for the effectiveness of heat treatment; a similar test is used for pasteurized milk when the enzyme phosphatase is destroyed by heat. Liquid whole egg and yolk should be pasteurized before drying. Imported liquid whole egg must also conform to the alpha-amylase test. Other nations pasteurize bulked egg also, but the processing times and temperatures vary.

TABLE 13. Salmonella from hens' eggs (shell). Historical record (excluding *S. pullorum* and *S. gallinarum*

Year	Country	Number examined	Number positive	Serotype
1947	England	166 (dirty shells)	9 (dirty shells)	*S. thompson*
		608 (clean shells)	1 (clean shells)	*S. thompson*
1950	USA	12 (bulked)	+	*S. paratyphi* B
1950	England	'Eggs' from one hen	+	*S. typhimurium*
1952	England	3,648	0	
1953	Australia	3,312	0	
1956	England	350 +	0	
1956	Japan	428	39	*S. give*
			26	*S. senftenberg*
1958	England	1,620	0	
1959	N. Ireland	60	1	*S. anatum*
1959	Japan	717	79	*S. senftenberg*
		(eggs unable to develop)		
1959	N. Ireland	'Eggs'	+	*S. infantis*
				S. albany
1959	England	12 (bulked in groups of 4)	+ (one group of 4)	*S. thompson*
1960	N. Ireland	150	4 (shells)	*S. typhimurium*
1960	England (Indian eggs)	24	1 (shell)	*S. enegal*

TABLE 14. Salmonella from egg products, 1961 and 1962

Egg products	1961			1962		
	Number examined	Number positive	Per cent	Number examined	Number positive	Per cent
Whole frozen	1,042	165	16	327	53	16
Whole dried	898	107	12	111	25	23
White frozen	675	41	6	187	35	19
White powder	214	18	8	103	28	27
White flake	536	68	13	236	44	19
Yolk dried	57	3	5	34	14	41
TOTAL	3,422	402	11	998	199	20

Liquid egg white coagulates at a lower temperature so that pasteurization is difficult but not impossible; a maximum temperature of 57·2 to 57·8 °C (135 to 136 °F) can be used, or higher if the egg white is stabilized in some way. Pan-dried flaked albumen may be heated in the dry state at 54·4°C (130°F) for 9 to 10 days to kill salmonellae but the treatment of spray-dried albumen by heat is unsatisfactory because of its low moisture content. It is hoped that in the future both these products will be made from pasteurized liquid albumen. The alpha-amylase test is not applicable to pasteurized egg white.

Irradiation of frozen liquid whole egg, or the white and yolk with small doses of gamma-rays will also kill salmonellae but the method is still without official sanction.

Desserts and sweets

In the sweet group, ice-cream, imitation cream, trifles, custards and other lightly cooked and uncooked milk and egg dishes and coconut confectionery have all been responsible for outbreaks of food poisoning.

Ice-cream

Ice-cream can now be regarded as a reasonably safe product in the UK, and the introduction of certain Regulations helped to bring about a big improvement in its hygienic quality.

The Ice-cream (Heat Treatment, etc.) Regulations of 1959, originally introduced in 1947, require ice-cream mix to be pasteurized by holding the mix either at 65·6°C (150°F) for at least 30 minutes, at 71·1°C (160°F) for at least 10 minutes or at 79·4°C

(175°F) for at least 15 seconds followed by cooling to 7·2°C (45°F) within 1½ hours and it must not rise above this temperature until it is frozen; it must remain frozen until sold. A mix which has been held at 149°C (300°F) for 2 seconds and transferred aseptically into sterile, airtight containers need not be reduced in temperature until required for freezing. This mix is distributed for use in the preparation of 'soft ice-cream' which is frozen at the counter immediately prior to sale.

'Soft ice-cream' is also prepared from the pasteurized mix stored at 7·2°C (45°F) until required for freezing at the counter. The responsibility for the hygienic handling of such unfrozen mixtures thus passes from the specialist manufacturer to those who may not be so conscious of the need for vigorous cleansing and sterilization of the freezer and other apparatus in contact with the ice-cream.

Ice-cream prepared with a cold-mix powder evaporated and dried from a liquid mix which has received approved heat treatment need not be heated again but must be frozen within an hour of reconstitution.

Before the Regulations were made, ice-cream mix was frozen at the convenience of the manufacturer and food-poisoning bacteria introduced by food handlers responsible for preparing the mix were sometimes provided with excellent conditions for growth prior to freezing; outbreaks are described in Chapters 6 and 8.

Another factor which has helped to improve the hygiene of the ice-cream trade is the introduction of a grading scheme based on tests for the bacteriological content of ice-cream samples. This method of control is used extensively in the UK. Competitive improvement between manufacturers has led to a general raising of the standard of cleanliness in other countries also.

It has been demonstrated frequently that thorough cleaning and disinfection of equipment is essential for the production of a high standard of bacterial cleanliness in ice-cream. The bacteriological examination of samples taken from different points throughout the processing plant will help to indicate sources of contamination arising from faults in cleaning procedures; sources or foci of contamination may be found in the cooler, in pipes or buckets used to convey the cream from the cooler to the ageing vat, or in the vat itself, freezer or conservator. Imperfect control of 'holder' type pasteurization may allow the survival of contaminants, from ingredients, which can multiply in imperfectly cleaned equipment. Various detergents are available for the preliminary washing process which should be followed by the application of steam, hypochlorite or other suitable bactericidal agent.

Imitation cream

Many outbreaks of salmonellosis and paratyphoid fever have been traced to the consumption of imitation cream cakes such as chocolate éclairs, cream buns, cream layer sponges, meringues and other confectionery including trifles garnished with cream.

The ingredients of the different types of confectionery cream vary widely. Usually they contain dried milk products emulsified with fat and a little sugar. Further nutriment is supplied from the choux pastry, sponge cakes and other confectionery in contact with the cream, and bacterial growth is encouraged.

Some creams have a high concentration of sugar and fat so that bacteria are unable to grow in them although they may survive for many days. Egg products are rarely incorporated into imitation cream but the food-poisoning organisms which may be present in liquid or dried egg products reach the cream from utensils, vessels, surfaces, hands and perhaps by splashes. It was assumed for many years that food-poisoning organisms originated from human excreters among food handlers responsible either for the manufacture of the cream or for its use in the bakery or kitchens. It is now known that, whilst there is always the possibility of infection from human sources, the first and more potent danger is the contamination of uncooked products such as cream by the salmonellae in the egg ingredients of cake and pastry mixes. The compulsory pasteurization of bulked whole egg has reduced, if not eliminated, the risk of paratyphoid fever and salmonella food poisoning from imitation cream cakes and other confectionery.

Bulked egg for drying can be, but is not always, pasteurized before dehydration. There is as yet no legislation in the United Kingdom for the pasteurization of egg albumen although many supplies are in fact heat treated before freezing or dehydration.

Fresh cream has largely superseded imitation cream; there are few outbreaks traced to fresh cream confectionery in the United Kingdom. Staphylococcal enterotoxin food poisoning from cream cakes is reported frequently in the United States of America but not in the United Kingdom.

Manufactured imitation cream is now pasteurized before canning and it is unusual to find a proprietary brand which is not of good bacteriological quality (low bacterial count) on delivery.

Outbreaks described in Chapter 6 illustrate the ease with which food-poisoning bacteria can spread from contaminated ingredients via mixing bowls, utensils and other articles to cream mixes and finished products; failure to disinfect piping and Savoy bags each time they are used is another factor in the spread of contamination.

Trifles, custards and other lightly cooked milk and egg dishes

All of these foods contain milk and egg constituents and so they are suitable for the growth of micro-organisms; they are mostly eaten cold so that there is often opportunity and time for bacterial multiplication after preparation.

Organisms from egg products are unlikely to survive the cooking but they may be introduced with bacteria from other ingredients such as sponge cakes contaminated from surfaces, utensils or fingers. There is no evidence for the survival of salmonellae in baked custards, custard tarts or flans, Swiss rolls or sponges. Moreover the results of experiments indicate that with normal baking procedures angel cake, Genoese slab, Japanese biscuits, macaroons and meringues are safe, but that when baking temperatures are allowed to fluctuate due to irregular opening of oven doors, salmonellae may survive. However, recontamination after cooking is considered to be the more serious hazard, particularly when powdered or flaked egg products are in use, because they are readily air-borne and dust-borne.

Coconut and gelatin

Desiccated coconut is frequently used to garnish and flavour cakes, trifles and other custard dishes. Many tons, graded according to the particle size, are imported annually into the UK for industrial use in cakes and biscuits, and for making sweets; it is used also by the housewife and canteen cook for cakes, puddings and desserts. In 1959 salmonellae including paratyphoid bacilli were isolated from 8 to 10 per cent of port samples of desiccated coconut. Cases of paratyphoid fever in children were traced to coconut confectionery and salmonellae including *S. paratyphi B* were isolated from sweetmeats and other confectionery coated with coconut. Industrial representation to the country of origin resulted in new legislation for improved hygiene which reduced the proportion of contaminated samples to negligible levels.

Salmonellae have been isolated from marshmallow as well as from uncooked coconut used as a coating. Occasional imports of gelatin used as a coagulant for marshmallow and for many other purposes have been found positive for salmonellae. Whether the organism survived the brief cooking of marshmallow or whether the cooked article became recontaminated in the whipping process was not known, but it was suspected that cooked mixtures may have been whipped in the same bowl as the cold uncooked mix. It is essential, therefore, to ensure that powdery commodities from food ingredients such as gelatin, coconut and egg are free from contamination with organisms of the salmonella group and staphylococci. Bacterial spores will survive in small numbers and it is almost impossible to eliminate them from dehydrated products. It is assumed that spores are eaten daily without harm, but when they germinate into bacilli which grow and multiply in rehydrated and cooked dishes there may be trouble.

Fish and other seafoods

Fish eaten freshly cooked is an improbable vehicle of bacterial food poisoning. Salmonellae are unlikely to be harboured in creatures with a low body temperature and mostly caught far out at sea. Nevertheless these organisms have been isolated from fish taken from polluted river water and also from fish taken from the holds of ships washed out with polluted dock water. Contamination may take place when the fish are gutted and filleted at the quayside or in shops. Made-up dishes such as fishcakes and fish pies may be contaminated with staphylococci from the hands of those working with cooked fish, cooked potatoes, batter and bread crumbs; there may be a build-up of contamination in equipment used for mashed potatoes, in the commercial production of fishcakes, so that a focus of infection is formed.

Clostridium botulinum type E may be found in some fish; whether the organism is a natural inhabitant of the fish-gut is not known. However, many outbreaks of botulism in Canada, the USA and Japan have been attributable to uncooked, or under-cooked, stale or fermented fish and also seal and whale meat. Smoked fish in open or vacuum packs, sold chilled or at ambient temperatures, and faults in canning of fish (tuna) have given rise to occasional outbreaks of botulism due to *Cl. botulinum* type E in various countries during recent years.

Food poisoning from *Vibrio parahaemolyticus* is common in Japan where fish and other seafoods may be infected from coastal waters.

Uncooked seafoods and also recontaminated cooked fish and crab meat have been reported as vehicles of infection.

Shell-fish

Oysters and mussels are often bred or fattened in the sewage-polluted waters of tidal estuaries, and oysters are usually consumed uncooked. From time to time cases and outbreaks of typhoid and paratyphoid fever are attributed to oysters collected from rivers receiving sewage from houses inhabited by carriers. The last outbreak of typhoid fever from this cause occurred in 1957.

There were four large stations in the United Kingdom for cleansing shell-fish, three for mussels and one for oysters. Of these only the Conway station survives; overhead expenses were great and stations cleansing mussels work only during the winter months; also, fisheries have failed. There are smaller stations for mussels from private fisheries and privately owned tanks for cleansing oysters; the water is usually purified by ultra-violet light. There are thirty or more of these small plants in the UK. They usually consist of a series of interconnected tanks; the water may be recirculated or continuously flowing from rivers or sea. The oysters are layed out on trays and remain in the tanks for 36 to 48 hours. Some of these stations may be ineffective, particularly when water is taken from highly polluted sources and the output of ultra-violet light is low. Organisms other than *Escherichia coli* and notably vibrio-type organisms can build up in the tanks and pipelines and also in the flesh of the oysters. Outbreaks of food poisoning have occurred from oysters treated in this way, although the agent of food poisoning is still not known.

At Conway the mussels brought by the fishermen are laid in large tanks and covered with freshly chlorinated sea-water for 48 hours. The mussels cleanse themselves by excretion and the internal contents drop through grids to the bottom of the tank. The cleansed shell-fish are bagged and collected by the fishermen (Fig. 9).

There are local laws relating to the cleansing of shell-fish. At Conway, for example, the Conway Mussel Fishery (Amendment) Order of 1948 states that any person taking mussels from the Conway River and failing 'to deposit them forthwith at the Purification Tanks' shall be guilty of an offence. On a more general scale there are over forty Closing Orders which prohibit the sale of shell-fish for food either absolutely or unless they have been treated in some way. These Orders are made under the Food and Drugs

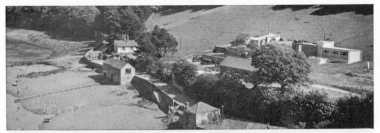

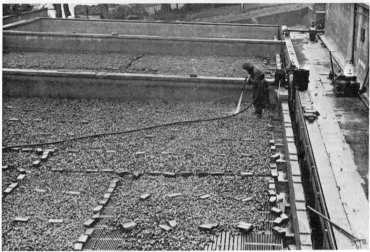

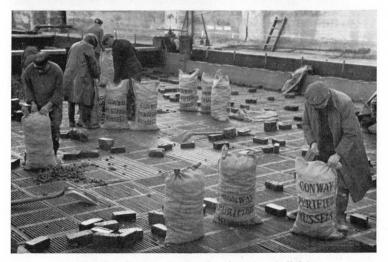

FIG. 9.   Conway Station for cleansing shell-fish

Act. They cover a large proportion of our coasts and of the areas suitable for growing shell-fish. If a fishery does not have a Closing Order there is probably no sewage pollution in the area or there is efficient treatment and the shell-fish fall regularly into the bacteriological Sanitary Grade I, that is, less than 5 *Esch. coli* per ml. of body tissue in 9 or 10 mussels or in single oysters. This standard is widely accepted in the United Kingdom and in Europe.

Closing Orders refer to the gathering, distribution, etc., of shell-fish for sale for human consumption, and so they do not prevent people from gathering them for their own consumption. The law is only broken when shell-fish are sold or otherwise distributed to other people. Thus, while it is not illegal for itinerant pickers to gather mussels from any shore, they may not legally sell them if they come from a Closed Area.

There are few recorded incidents of bacterial food poisoning from mussels, since they are usually cooked by the consumer. The cockle industry is different. The cockles are collected into huts, cooked and sometimes salted before distribution. Incidents thought to have been caused by cockles have occurred during warm weather when bacterial multiplication after cooking, during storage and retail sale in shops and on stalls, will be greatest.

From 1964 onwards particular attention has been given to outbreaks of gastroenteritis of recognizable aetiology following the eating of oysters which have been cleaned in tanks of water treated with ultra-violet light. The *Esch. coli* count of samples of oysters associated with outbreaks is usually satisfactory but counts of other organisms may be high. The well-known agents of food poisoning have not been found either in the oysters or in the stools of patients. The isolation of *V. parahaemolyticus* in some coastal waters and sea creatures has suggested that vibrios may be responsible for the oyster disease.

Shell-fish imported from other countries should be accompanied by a certificate of bacterial purity.

Frozen cooked seafoods

Frozen cooked prawns, shrimps, and lobster tails are produced by a number of countries for international trade. They may be handled extensively after cooking and before freezing yet for most imports there have been few isolations of salmonellae from samples examined directly from the port. It must be assumed therefore that they are rarely contaminated by human excreters and that they are not a natural source of salmonellae. Even raw frozen samples are rarely positive for salmonellae.

Staphylococci, from the hands of workers, are found more frequently, although outbreaks of staphylococcal food poisoning from seafoods are not common in the United Kingdom. *V. parahaemolyticus* may be isolated from imported frozen cooked prawns, and the implication of prawn cocktails in food poisoning due to this vibrio is suspected; other pathogenic vibrios have been found also.

Tentative microbiological standards for the guidance of manufacturers and port health authorities have been of value in producing a more hygienic product. Viable counts of less than 100,000 per g are the rule; recommendations that there should be not more than 20 per g of coliform bacilli and not more than 100 to 1,000 per g of coagulase-positive staphylococci are readily attainable with care in manufacture.

The responsibility of maintaining the product in a good bacteriological condition rests with the user; as for frozen foods in general, the time and temperature of storage between thawing and consumption are important.

Fruit

Acid fruits, for example cooked or canned apples and plums alone or in tarts and cordials, will not allow the growth of pathogenic bacteria but the organisms may survive for indefinite periods of time. It is advisable to wash dessert fruit, such as grapes and plums which are not normally peeled before eating, in water containing a small amount of sodium hypochlorite so that the amount of available chlorine in solution is approximately 60 to 80 p.p.m. (the actual dilution of the product will depend on its concentration of hypochlorite and the volume of water used for washing). Many kinds of dessert fruits are imported from countries where the rate of excretion of intestinal pathogens is high and where the fly plays a major role in the spread of infection.

Vegetables

Freshly cooked vegetables may be regarded as safe but it is wise to wash salad vegetables such as lettuce, tomatoes, radishes, cucumber, and watercress in water with added sodium hypochlorite (60 to 80 p.p.m. available chlorine) as recommended for dessert fruit.

In 1959 a small outbreak of food poisoning was attributed to an excess of the alkaloid solanine in the skin of imported potatoes. Solanine poisoning is uncommon, but outbreaks have been described in other countries due to unusually high concentrations of solanine developing in the skin or green shoots of potatoes.

Pickles, sauces and mayonnaise

Pickles, sauces and mayonnaise made with vinegar are highly acid and they are unlikely to cause food poisoning. Certain bacteria can grow in acid foods and some of these are able to cause spoilage, but they are not dangerous for man. Dressings and sauces made without vinegar, such as Hollandaise sauce, may contain eggs, fat and flavouring matter only. As they are highly suitable for bacterial growth, they should be prepared with great care and attention to hygiene and they should be eaten within 1 or, at the most, 2 hours of preparation, unless stored in the refrigerator.

Some countries like a bland mayonnaise with a pH of 5 to 7; others, such as the UK, prefer a sharp flavour and add vinegar or lemon juice until the pH is approximately 3 to 4·5 and the growth of pathogens repressed. When mayonnaise has a neutral pH, salmonellae from eggs or staphylococci from man can grow and many outbreaks of food poisoning from this commodity have been reported. Ingredients of uncooked non-acid foods should not include ducks' eggs or unpasteurized hen egg products.

Powdered foods

Dried food substances are not sterile. Some micro-organisms and particularly spores survive dehydration, but they will not grow until water is added and the temperature is suitable.

Proprietary cake mixes and meringue powders which incorporate unpasteurized powdered egg products may contain organisms of the salmonella group. Outbreaks of salmonellosis following the use of contaminated cake mixes have been described in Canada and the USA. Dried milk contaminated with salmonellae caused an interstate outbreak of salmonella food poisoning in the USA; 17 families were affected. The source of contamination was thought to be raw milk from one of 800 farms supplying the dehydration plant. Milled products such as wheat and other cornflours and also rice may contain sporing organisms such as *Bacillus cereus*. Cornflour sauce and cooked rice have been vehicles of food poisoning due to this organism. This and other sporing organisms are frequent contaminants of dairy plants and may cause spoilage.

Spices, dehydrated soups, baby foods and other convenience foods will all contain spores but they should be low in numbers.

Fats

Lard, margarine, butter and other fats do not encourage the growth of pathogenic bacteria, and they may be disregarded as media for food-poisoning organisms. If they are contaminated during preparation with typhoid, paratyphoid or dysentery bacilli, then small numbers, surviving for many days, may cause infection. An unusual outbreak occurred in the USA from staphylococcal enterotoxin in butter emulsified in milk.

Bread

Many people are worried about the contamination of bread, and they regard the handling of unwrapped loaves with concern. Bread is seldom if ever responsible for bacterial food poisoning; the crust forms a barrier against the invasion of bacteria and, furthermore, the substance of the loaf is far too dry to allow the growth of bacteria unless it is in contact with a moist foodstuff. Intestinal pathogens causing infection in small doses only may be transferred on sliced bread from the hands of an excreter to the victim.

It is a matter of common observation that moulds grow readily on stale bread or on bread wrapped too soon after baking, but hitherto the growth of moulds in bread has not been regarded as a hazard.

Bread 'ropy' from the prolific growth of aerobic spore bearers has been described as a cause of food poisoning overseas.

Jam and similar sweetstuffs

Among those foods which may be disregarded as vehicles of food poisoning are the preserves such as jam, and also honey and syrup; they usually contain 60 per cent or more of sugar which will not permit the survival of most bacteria. Moulds may grow on the top of jam, especially when the sugar concentration is lower than required for preservation. Moulds have not been recorded as a cause of food poisoning but when the mycelium of certain fungi grow throughout a food substance there may be danger from mycotoxins. Little is known about the pathological effect of these toxins on man but in certain animals and in fish they have been shown to cause liver damage.

6

Examples of Outbreaks of Food Poisoning

The occurrence of bacterial food poisoning depends on a peculiar set of circumstances; the following essential factors must be present:

1. The infecting organism (causal agent), which has reached the kitchen in foodstuffs or which is present in the food handler or in animals.
2. The hands of the food handler or kitchen surfaces, utensils, boards, cloths and other articles of equipment soiled by contaminated foods or hands.
3. A food suitable for bacterial growth.
4. Conditions favourable for warm storage over a period of 2 hours or more.
5. Susceptible human subjects.

The investigation of food poisoning depends on the ability to find out the details relating to each of these five factors. In Britain, food poisoning is a notifiable disease under the Food and Drugs Act, 1955, and the local medical officer of health must be informed of all cases and outbreaks. The investigation is then a matter for medical and health officers, microbiologists and epidemiologists. The sooner an outbreak is notified to the authorities the greater the chance of isolating the germs responsible for the outbreak from the patient's stool and perhaps vomit, and of obtaining the remains of the contaminated foodstuff.

In a group of people, some of whom fall ill, the proof of food poisoning depends on the isolation of the food-poisoning organisms from a foodstuff common to all the patients and also from the stools of a number of patients, particularly when the nature of the outbreak suggests that salmonellae are the causal agents. The character of the causal agent and its behaviour in food may indicate the reason for its growth in food and indicate the preventive measures which must be taken.

The collection of relevant information about the clinical nature of the outbreak, incubation period, numbers affected, those at risk, and the type of food suspected, is also most important if the original source of the organism is to be found and the faults in production corrected.

The clinical symptoms and incubation period, as described in Chapter 3, will generally indicate whether the illness is due to the toxin or infection type of bacterial food poisoning. An important part of the inquiry is to find out the foods eaten in common by all the patients, and the foods eaten by those who remained well, although it must be remembered that not all those at risk through eating the contaminated meal will necessarily feel ill.

Immediately information about food poisoning is received, the kitchen staff should be warned not to throw any foodstuffs away. The cause of many food-poisoning incidents has been obscured because left-over remains of meats have been discarded before the health inspector arrived.

The isolation and identification of bacteria of known pathogenic significance from the food and the patients is the key to further investigation. It may also bring to light contaminated sources of raw materials, imported or home-produced, which will require further investigation and research to make them safe.

The food vehicle is often found among prepared meats and poultry, warmed-up dishes, lightly cooked egg and milk products, and other foods which are suitable for bacterial growth and which may have been left for some hours without refrigeration.

If the suspected foodstuff is not available for examination then it may be useful to sample the ingredients, particularly raw meats and poultry which are known to be sources of salmonellae.

If the nature of the outbreak suggests that it is due to salmonellae other than *Salmonella typhi*, then enquiries should be made about all raw meat and poultry and other protein foods used in the kitchen and samples examined from kitchen, retail and wholesale sources. Stools from patients and food handlers must be examined also.

If food poisoning from staphylococcal enterotoxin is suspected, stools and vomit samples from patients should be examined as well as foods, and also swabs from nose, throat, hands and any pustular spots or even healed lesions on food handlers. The results may reveal food handlers carrying the staphylococcus which has grown and produced enterotoxin in the food.

When *Clostridium welchii* food poisoning is suspected, food and stools from patients must be examined. The organism is common in many foodstuffs and it is excreted in small numbers by most people. Thus there is little or no significance in positive results from food handlers. Efforts should be directed towards obtaining better cooling and cold storage facilities.

Whatever the source of the food poisoning bacteria, faults in preparation and storage will have led to multiplication of the organism in the cooked food (or vehicle) which is the immediate cause of the outbreak. Efforts should be made, therefore, to find out not only the source but also how the organisms spread from raw to cooked foods or from persons to cooked foods in relation to methods of food preparation and where the time lag occurred after cooking which allowed growth at temperatures convenient for the organism.

It cannot be assumed that food handlers found to be excreting the relevant organism after an outbreak are necessarily the source of infection; they may be victims through handling or eating raw materials already contaminated before entering the kitchen. Nevertheless, such victims with loose stools may help to spread infection to foods and in the environment.

Examples of typical food-poisoning outbreaks are given in the next few pages. In the first, a straightforward outbreak of staphylococcal toxin food poisoning, the chain of events could easily have been broken if those responsible for the preparation of the food had understood the factors causing the contamination and had taken steps to ensure efficient cold storage.

The ham sandwich outbreak (Fig. 10)

A coach-load of people left London one summer morning on their way to the coast for a day's outing. They took with them, for their lunch, ham sandwiches cut and prepared at a public house in the home area. Before they had travelled far many had started to eat their sandwiches, and as they were nearing the coast the first victim began to feel ill; soon other members of the party were unwell. When they arrived at the coast the illness was acute and several people were taken into the local hospitals.

News of the outbreak soon reached the medical officer of health for the area, and the coach was searched for the remains of the food; fortunately, one or two ham sandwiches were found. Specimens of stool and vomit were collected from the patients who had been taken to hospital, and these specimens were submitted to the local public health laboratory. The following day investigations were started by the medical officer of health in London. Inquiries were

made at the public house where the sandwiches had been prepared; those responsible for making them were questioned about the
method of preparation and the source of the ham. The bacteriologists at the coast town found large numbers of staphylococci
in ham from the sandwiches retrieved from the coach, and

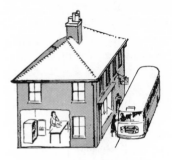

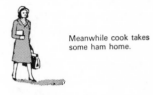

Meanwhile cook takes
some ham home.

Ham, contaminated with cook's
nasal staphylococci and stored
in a broken refrigerator, made into
sandwiches for a coach party.

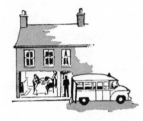

She and husband taken
to hospital that night.

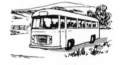

Some were eaten on the way.

At the seaside several of the
party taken to hospital.

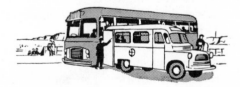

FIG. 10.   The ham sandwich outbreak on a trip to the seaside

LABORATORY FINDINGS
Staphylococci of the same type isolated from ham, faeces, vomit, and from nose
of cook.

COMMENTS
1. Food handlers must not finger their noses.
2. Food must be stored in a refrigerator below 4°C (39·2°F).

staphylococci were found in the vomit and faeces of the patients who were in hospital. At the same time another laboratory found staphylococci in the remains of the ham taken from the public house. When the staphylococci from the three sources were compared, they were found to belong to the same type—one often associated with foodstuffs known to have caused staphylococcal enterotoxin food poisoning. The woman who prepared the sandwiches took home a small portion of the ham to share with her husband for supper; about 2 hours later they, too, became violently ill and were taken to hospital by ambulance. The strains of staphylococci isolated from these patients proved to be of the same type as that isolated from the specimens examined in the coast town and in London. The next step was to discover how these organisms had reached the meat, and why they had multiplied.

The ham was cooked at the public house; it was stored in a refrigerator and brought out day by day for the preparation of sandwiches. There were two faults: the first that the worker used her hands freely to hold the ham bone and the sliced ham, and second that the refrigerator motor failed so that conditions were warm inside the cabinet. The particular staphylococcus was resident in the nose of the worker and it would frequently be on her hands, and pass from her hands to the ham. Conditions were ideal for multiplication—warm summer weather and lack of refrigeration. Staphylococci grow well and produce toxin in many cured meats because they can tolerate salt. There were many millions per gram in the ham, and the rapid onset of violent symptoms indicated the presence of a high concentration of toxin. The organisms were isolated also from samples of faeces and vomit from the patients.

It is worth noting that the carrier herself was a victim of the toxin formed by the organisms transferred from her nose to the ham. Immunity to the powerful toxin which certain staphylococci produce during active multiplication in foodstuffs is not acquired while the organism is resident in the nose or throat. It is not easy to remove the organism; in some instances it may be possible, but in others it is better for the carrier to be transferred to other work. It may not be possible to eliminate staphylococci from the hands even after washing.

The contaminated glaze outbreak (Fig. 11)

In another widespread outbreak of food poisoning due to staphylococcal toxin, the glaze on the outside of liver sausage

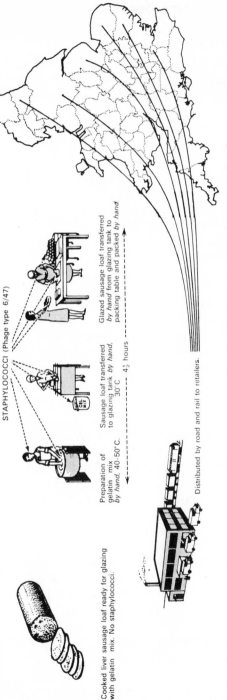

STAPHYLOCOCCI (Phage type 6/47)

Cooked liver sausage loaf ready for glazing with gelatin mix. No staphylococci.

Preparation of gelatin mix *by hand*. 40–50°C.

Sausage loaf transferred to glazing tank *by hand*. 30°C

Glazed sausage loaf transferred *by hand* from glazing tank to packing table and packed *by hand*

◄─────── 4½ hours ───────►

Distributed by road and rail to retailers.

Fig. 11. The contaminated glaze outbreak of food poisoning—staphylococcal toxin

LESSONS LEARNT FROM OUTBREAK

1. All contact of hands with food should be avoided.

2. Personnel with septic fingers or other skin sepsis, acute colds, or abdominal upsets with diarrhoea, should not engage in food handling. The nose is the reservoir of staphylococci and infection may be conveyed from nose to food via the hands.

3. Hands must be washed frequently while handling food, and particularly after visiting the WC. There should be hot running water, antiseptic soap and plentiful supplies of clean towels, or preferably destructible paper towels or an enclosed roller towel.

4. All cooked foods and made-up foodstuffs including fillings and glazes intended to be eaten cold should be given sufficient heat treatment to render them sterile or free from vegetative bacteria. Surplus filling and glazing material should not be stored overnight.

5. Cooked foods, not intended for immediate consumption, should be wrapped or covered and kept at a temperature not higher than 4°C (39·2°F).

6. Food containers and utensils should be well washed in hot water containing a good detergent and rinsed in water as hot as possible (not less than 80°C). A disinfectant, e.g. hypochlorite, used separately or combined with the detergent is an advantage.

7. Food containers and utensils, after rinsing in hot water 80–90°C (176–194°F), should be allowed to drain and not be dried with a cloth. Where it is essential to wipe them, paper may be used or cloths should be washed daily.

loaves became heavily contaminated with staphylococci of a food-poisoning type. This foodstuff was prepared on a large scale by a factory, and the meat loaves were distributed over a wide area of the country. More than 400 cases were reported in this outbreak, and there may have been many hundreds more which remained unnotified.

Large numbers of specimens of the liver sausage loaf were sent to the laboratory from various parts of the country, and each specimen told the same story. The glaze contained up to 100 million per g of staphylococci, whereas the meat part of the loaf was almost free from organisms. It was clear that the loaf had been correctly processed, that it was free from contamination, and that the glaze only had been contaminated during preparation.

The factory was visited and the methods of manufacture were watched closely. At the same time swabs were taken from the nose, hands and any lesions or spots of all the personnel engaged in the processing, glazing or packing. Table tops and utensils were also swabbed and samples of glaze and the constituents were taken for examination; faults in the methods of production were observed. The operative, his shirt-sleeves rolled up to the elbow, blended each ingredient by hand in a steam-jacketed container; the temperature of the mix never rose above 50°C (122°F) so that contaminating organisms from the hands would not be killed at any stage in the preparation.

The process of glazing took several hours; a jug was continually filled by hand from the tank and the glaze was poured over the minced liver loaves resting on grids above the tank. The bulk supply of glaze was kept in the large jacketed container while the glazing was in progress, and the small tank which supplied the well for glazing was replenished when necessary from the bulk supply, kept at approximately 34°C (93·2°F).

The outbreak took place during a warm spell of weather in June, when conditions were ideal for the multiplication of the contaminating staphylococci. The glaze was an excellent medium for bacterial growth, and supplies left over from one day's work were kept overnight in the refrigerator to be added to the fresh batch of glaze made the following day, thus serving as an inoculum.

The visit to the factory took place one week after the outbreak had occurred. By this time the food-poisoning staphylococcus was fairly widespread in the glazing and packing room. It was found in the nose and on the hands of four people, and in swabs from portions of equipment and the paper used for packing the meat loaves. After outbreaks of food-borne disease the organisms responsible may become more widely dispersed in the environment than hitherto. There are many means of spread of infection including the handling of communal utensils and other equipment, and the use of communal roller towels. It is advisable to take series of specimens from the nose, throat and hands of suspected carriers, in order to distinguish transient from persistent carriage.

In this particular outbreak the follow-up work revealed that the employee who prepared the glaze harboured in his nose the type of staphylococcus which caused the outbreak. He was transferred to other work which did not involve the handling of susceptible foodstuffs. It was agreed that the glazing operation should be stopped temporarily and the particular area of the factory was thoroughly cleaned and disinfected.

The methods used were wrong and in order to minimize the risk of further contamination, it was recommended that the hands of the operatives should not come in open contact with the glaze during or after preparation, and that after the ingredients had been added the glaze mix would be brought to the boil. It was suggested that glazing should be carried out in a cool room and that the temperature of the glaze during this process should be maintained at approximately 60 °C (140 °F); any glaze left over after the day's work would be discarded. Thus a build-up of bacteria in the glaze would be prevented.

The lambs' tongues outbreak (Fig. 12)

An outbreak of food poisoning which occurred in a factory canteen was due to the contamination of lambs' tongues with staphylococci from the hands of two members of the kitchen staff. The frozen tongues arrived in sacks. They were allowed to thaw; they were then cooked, and laid out carefully in rows on enamel trays which stood on a table in the kitchen until the tongues were cool enough to handle. Six people stood around the table and removed the skin from each tongue, using hand and knife. The skinned tongues were again placed in rows on enamel trays and allowed to stand in the kitchen for a further period, before refrigeration overnight. Early next morning they were taken out and sliced by one man. The slices were placed on dinner plates which were kept warm in the hotplate container until ready for lunch at midday.

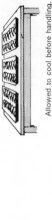
Frozen lambs' tongues arrived in sacks.

Boiled for 2½ hours.

Allowed to cool before handling.

Infected tongues allowed to cool for about two hours before going into refrigerator. Staphylococci multiply.

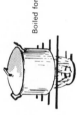
Six people helped to skin the tongues by hand. Two were found to be hand carriers of food-poisoning staphylococci.

42°C
60°C
145°C

Plates of sliced tongue placed in hot-plate for one to two hours before serving. Staphylococci multiply in food on top shelf (42°C).

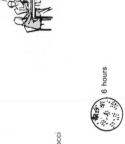
CANTEEN
70 people ill after eating tongue. Incubation period — three hours.

Next morning tongues taken from refrigerator and sliced by hand. Opportunity for further contamination.

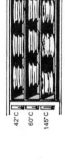

2 hours   4 hours   6 hours

Staphylococci growing in tongue as seen microscopically at intervals after handling.

FIG. 12.   The lambs' tongues outbreak of food poisoning—staphylococcal toxin

It was shown that, although the lower two shelves of the hot cupboard were maintained at a temperature which would kill most bacteria, the temperature of the top shelf was much lower, in fact suitable for bacterial multiplication. A few cooked tongues not used for the meal were stored in the refrigerator. They were examined at the laboratory and found to contain large numbers of staphylococci of the usual food-poisoning type.

The large factory canteen was visited a few days after the outbreak to investigate the source of the staphylococci and the reason for their multiplication.

Many people worked in the kitchen, and nose and hand swabs were taken from all of them. Table tops, floors and other places were swabbed and samples of dust were collected.

Staphylococci were isolated from swabs of table tops and from dust even after instructions had been carried out that all surfaces should be cleaned with detergent and disinfected with hypochlorite solution. The tables were wooden and it seemed impossible to eliminate bacteria from the nooks and crannies of the irregular surface. The staphylococcus was found on the hands of two of the staff who had helped to skin the tongues; nose and hand swabs were taken at weekly intervals for several months. The organism was persistently cultured from the hands although there was no evidence that it was present in the nose. Finally, when drastic measures were used, such as exposure to ultra-violet light and the application of flavine to the hands, negative swabs were obtained. In the meantime, neither person was allowed to handle food known to encourage the growth of bacteria. The skinning by hand of cooked tongues while they are still warm always introduces a hazard of contamination by staphylococci. Outbreaks of staphylococcal food poisoning have occurred from large cooked tongues also. The long slow cooling of the cooked tongue followed by storage in the press provide admirable conditions for multiplication. There will be no further cooking when the tongue is eaten cold so that neither the organism nor its toxin will be destroyed. In the canning process of sterilization both the organism and its toxin are eliminated. Home processing should include a further cook after pressing.

Poisoned ice-cream

The Ice-Cream (Heat Treatment, etc.) Regulations introduced in 1947 stipulate that liquid ice-cream mix must be pasteurized and immediately cooled to 7·2°C (45°F) within 1½ hours of heat treatment. The chance contamination of ice-cream by excreters of intestinal pathogens, nasal and hand carriers of staphylococci and other nose and throat organisms capable of causing disease was far greater before the Regulations than at present. There was time for contaminating organisms to multiply in the mix before it was heated or after heating before it was frozen, and thus outbreaks of infection and toxin poisoning occurred. In 1945, for instance, staphylococci carried in the nose and on the hands of a worker in the cook-house of an army hospital were introduced into batches of ice-cream mix after the ingredients had been cooked. The mix was allowed to cool slowly overnight and 20 to 30 hours elapsed before freezing. The staphylococci multiplied abundantly and formed enough harmful toxin to affect some 700 people. Had the mix been frozen very soon after it had been cooked, as required by the present Regulations, there would have been no opportunity for the organisms to multiply, the toxin would not have been formed and the food poisoning would not have occurred.

The typhoid outbreak at Aberystwyth (1947) described in Chapter 8 followed the contamination of ice-cream mix, several hours before freezing, by a urinary excreter of *Salmonella typhi*.

Cheese outbreaks

In the spring of 1944 a family outbreak of staphylococcal toxin food poisoning followed the consumption of cheese made from goats' milk; it was the first of its kind to be reported in this country. Of six people, the five who became acutely ill 4 to 5 hours after tea had all eaten cheese made from goats' milk; the sixth, who escaped illness, had not eaten the cheese. Samples of this cheese showed the presence of many millions of staphylococci per gram and the same type of staphylococcus was found in the faeces of one of the patients. This cheese was made by adding rennet to fresh goats' milk; the whey was strained through a clean muslin bag and the cheese pressed into shape. Throat, nose and hand swabs from those concerned in the milking and the cheese making failed to reveal staphylococci and there were no lesions on the hands of the milker or on the udders or teats of the goats. Yet from the freshly drawn milk of one goat the same type of staphylococcus was isolated, and it was assumed that multiplication of the organisms had taken place in the milk. Furthermore, extracts of the staphylococci isolated from the cheese produced violent symptoms in a human volunteer.

Some unusual outbreaks of staphylococcal food poisoning from Cheddar cheese drew attention to the fact that milk contaminated with staphylococci from the cow and insufficiently heated to kill the organisms could introduce staphylococci at the start of cheese making. If traces of penicillin or other antibiotic used in the treatment of cows suffering from staphylococcal and streptococcal diseases are present in milk, then the starter culture used for fermentation may be suppressed and the staphylococcus encouraged to grow in its place.

Such cheeses are mostly second grade and used only for processing, but they have sometimes been eaten and caused sickness. It is by no means certain that this cheese would be safe after processing. It has been recommended therefore that all milk intended for cheese making should be pasteurized and a law to this effect has already been passed in New Zealand. Nearly every year there are one or more outbreaks of staphylococcal food poisoning from milk which has not been pasteurized. Although this milk may be designated TT it can nevertheless be contaminated with food-poisoning organisms from the cow, milker or equipment.

The spoiled pressed beef

The following account of an outbreak of food poisoning due to contaminated pressed beef provides a further illustration of the difficulty of satisfactorily disinfecting wooden table tops.

The outbreak occurred in a central factory responsible for distributing open-pack pressed meat of various types to subsidiary firms in different countries. Complaints had been received that the meat packs were arriving at their destination not only softened with liquefied gelatin but that they had caused mild food poisoning symptoms. The complaints had continued for some weeks before the laboratory was asked to investigate the trouble. The manufacture of the pressed meat was watched from the beginning to end, specimens were taken, and from the bacteriological results the following story was pieced together.

The meat, often of a poor quality, arrived frozen; it was allowed to thaw, and cut up into convenient portions on a large wooden table in a room which also contained boilers. The meat was then placed in the brine tanks built into a corridor leading from the work-room. After some days in the pickle solution the meat was removed on to the wooden table, and later transferred to the boilers. It was cooked for 2 hours, and then allowed to cool on the same wooden table, cut up into small pieces and placed in the press tins by hand. When each tin was packed, a solution of gelatin was poured over the meat and a lid pressed down by means of a clamp. The cans of meat were allowed to cool slowly overnight in an adjoining room.

Specimens examined in the laboratory revealed that the organism responsible for the liquefaction of the gelatin was *Proteus*; it was found on the wooden table, in the brine tank and in several specimens of cooked meat. This organism is widely distributed in nature, and whatever its origin it had established itself in the wooden crevices of the working table.

The solution in the brine tank contained approximately 6 per cent of sodium chloride which was far below the recommended strength; thus the organisms, instead of being inhibited, were able to thrive in large numbers. When chunks of pickled meat were taken from the brine tank and allowed to rest on the wooden table, the contaminated salt solution seeped into the rough surface, and the infecting organism remained in the cracks in spite of thorough washing, scrubbing and the recommended treatment with chlorine solution. The cooked meat coming straight from the boilers was bacteriologically sterile, but it was soon contaminated with *Proteus* from the table, and also no doubt from the hands of the operatives. Unaware of the dangers, the workers placed both hands on the surface of the meat and gelatin mix in the closely packed tins in order to press the meat well down before applying the lid. The warm meat coated with gelatin was stored at atmospheric temperature overnight and provided an ideal medium for bacterial growth; it was not surprising therefore that the gelatin had started to liquefy by the time the packs had reached their destination.

Two main recommendations were given. The first was to replace the wooden table by one with a hard impervious surface, which could be easily cleaned and used exclusively for cutting up the cooked meat into pieces for the press tin; a chopping block or other wooden surface was considered essential for carving up the freshly thawed meat. It seemed possible also to transfer the chunks of meat straight from the brine tanks to the boilers without resting them on the table. The second recommendation was to increase the strength of the brine in the pickle tank in order to discourage the survival of the spoilage organisms. Also it was explained to the employees that bacteria causing spoilage and food poisoning could be transferred from raw meat to cooked meat by hands and that those workers handling cooked meats should be particularly careful to wash their hands immediately before commencing work.

The pressed beef outbreaks (Fig. 13)

A group of outbreaks due to staphylococcal toxin food poisoning from contaminated pressed beef are of interest because they illustrate once again the danger which may arise from much-handled cooked meat allowed to cool slowly overnight at atmospheric temperature.

During a warm summer, four outbreaks of food poisoning were reported almost simultaneously. At first, there seemed no connection between them; one had occurred on an express train speeding North, another at a wedding party held at an east coast town, another at a south coast resort, and the last in London. Specimens of food soon began to arrive at the laboratory; they included pressed beef which had been eaten by those affected in all four outbreaks. Large numbers of staphylococci of the usual food-poisoning type were isolated from many samples of pressed beef. In the meantime, the medical officer of health and health inspectors of the local authorities concerned had traced the origin of the various supplies to one particular factory. The factory was owned by a well-established and reputable firm of food manufacturers, who were astonished at the suggestion that they might have been responsible for any carelessness in production methods. Nevertheless, they co-operated willingly, genuinely anxious to find the cause of the trouble.

As usual the process of manufacture was watched from beginning to end. Samples of meat were collected at every stage of manufacture of the pressed beef, together with nose and hand swabs from all those in any way connected with its production; swabs from tables, utensils, and press cans were also taken. The laboratory results showed that the toxin-producing strain of staphylococcus was present in specimens of meat only after they had been handled in the process of filling the press cans, and the chef who was responsible for this procedure was the only member of the staff who was carrying the infecting organisms on his hands. He had been doing this work for many years, and it was assumed that he had only recently become a hand carrier of a food-poisoning type of staphylococcus. It may be difficult to convince carriers of potentially pathogenic bacteria of the part that they may play in the spread of infection.

The brine tank contained salt solution of the correct strength

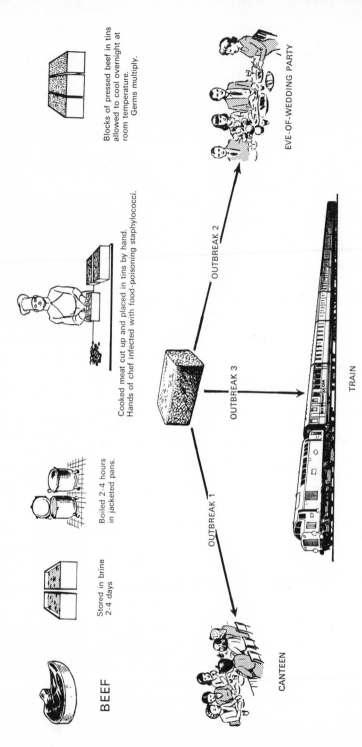

Blocks of pressed beef in tins allowed to cool overnight at room temperature. Germs multiply.

Cooked meat cut up and placed in tins by hand. Hands of chef infected with food-poisoning staphylococci.

Boiled 2-4 hours in jacketed pans.

Stored in brine 2-4 days

BEEF

EVE-OF-WEDDING PARTY

OUTBREAK 2

OUTBREAK 3

TRAIN

OUTBREAK 1

CANTEEN

FIG. 13. Pressed beef outbreaks of food poisoning—staphylococcal toxin

(16 to 18 per cent) and no staphylococci were found in it, nor were these organisms isolated from the samples of raw meat examined; samples of meat taken directly from the boiler were practically sterile. Only the chef's hands and the utensils used by him yielded the toxin-producing staphylococcus. His hands and nose were swabbed for many weeks; the hands were invariably positive, a few staphylococci were found in the nose on one occasion only. Many ways were tried to rid the hands of the staphylococci without success; the organisms still remained after washing.

The problem was temporarily solved by a change in the method of manufacture of the pressed beef, which was pressed into cans, hermetically sealed and heat treated. The cans were later discarded when it was desired to dispense the beef in open packs.

Other staphylococcal outbreaks

Many family outbreaks of staphylococcal food poisoning are caused simply by the contamination of cooked meats such as ham and similar products by the hands of food handlers in shops and homes, followed by lack of care in keeping these products cold during storage so that multiplication of the organisms and toxin production are encouraged.

The foods at wedding receptions are notorious vehicles of staphylococcal food poisoning. For example, 40 of 139 guests at a wedding developed vomiting, abdominal pain and diarrhoea about 2 hours after a meal which included turkey and ham. Identical strains of staphylococci were isolated from turkey and ham, and from septic spots on the hand as well as from the nose of the food handler who had cut the ham and turkey the night before the reception.

At a dog show on a hot day, 30 of 120 spectators who ate cold chicken and salad for lunch developed abdominal pain, diarrhoea and vomiting 2 to 3 hours later; 14 were admitted to hospital. The cooked chickens were left at 'tent' temperature overnight and jointed the following morning. There were 55 million per g of staphylococci in a pooled sample of chicken joints.

Beef, ham and tongue, remnants of a meal eaten in a church hall, were found to contain millions per g of staphylococci after all of 38 elderly ladies complained of symptoms; 11 were hospitalized. The meats had been handled by a number of persons including a chef, responsible for the slicing, who had recently returned to work after three weeks' absence with an injured finger and tonsillitis. There were no obvious lesions on his hands.

Counts of *Staphylococcus aureus* from 18 to 200 million per g were found in vanilla cakes eaten by five families who reported sickness, abdominal pain and in some instances diarrhoea 3 to 6 hours later. The cakes were sold from market stalls on a hot day. Staphylococci were also grown from a metal mixing bowl, an old burn on the hand of a bakery worker and from the eczematous lesions on the right hand and elbow of another bakery worker; both were involved in the preparation of the vanilla cakes.

In all these instances the enterotoxin responsible for illness was demonstrated in growth from the staphylococci and sometimes from the food itself.

Cold chicken is so frequently responsible for staphylococcal food poisoning, it is worthwhile to consider the reasons and to describe the events in the kitchen preceding such outbreaks.

Doctors at a lunch party were taken ill 2 to 4 hours after their meal of cold chicken and salad. The chicken had been cooked the day before and dismembered by hand while still warm. The portions were piled on trays and eventually placed in the refrigerator overnight. The cooling rate was slow and staphylococci from the hands of the workers were quick to grow in the warm chicken flesh. Multiplication would continue when the chicken was removed from the cold room and before service. A similar outbreak occurred on an aircraft after a meal of cold chicken prepared in the same way. The main fault was in portioning the chicken while still warm. The carcasses should not have been touched until cold and required for service. When food is cold the staphylococci will be slow to grow and the numbers will remain low until consumption if this is soon after the poultry carcasses have been portioned.

Food handlers should be aware that staphylococci are commonly present on the skin of the hands and other parts of the body; washing by ordinary means in soap and water does not remove them. Thus, care in handling cooked foods and, above all, care in prompt and persistent cold storage is essential. Small numbers are harmless but, as they grow, toxin is formed in the food and the longer the storage out of a refrigerator the larger the number of staphylococci and the greater the volume of toxin.

Canned foods

Although canned goods should normally be regarded as safe, there have been instances in which leakage after processing has given rise to staphylococcal and salmonella food poisoning; even typhoid bacilli have multiplied in canned meat after leakage through microscopic holes.

In a series of outbreaks arising from 2·72 kg (6 lb) cans of peas it was found that the employee handling the cans after the water-cooling process had septic lesions on her hands caused by a food-poisoning strain of staphylococcus. A very occasional can was imperfect in its construction and a small pinhole in a seam would allow staphylococci from her hands to be sucked in with water while the can was still under vacuum—the pressure being lower inside than outside. The staphylococci grew inside the can and produced toxin but not gas so that the spoiled cans were not blown and there was no indication that the contents were contaminated. The degree of heat necessary to cook canned peas would be insufficient to destroy the toxin.

Similar outbreaks have been known to occur from freshly opened cans of meat, particularly corned beef, and again contaminated cooling water or contamination from the hands of employees were suspected as the source of the organism growing inside the can. A similar method of contamination may occur with organisms of the salmonella group including typhoid bacilli (Chapter 8).

Some canned meats such as ham, pork and veal in large containers are not given sufficient heat treatment to sterilize, in a deliberate attempt to produce a more appetizing food. The following incident illustrates the hazard which may occur.

The contaminated ham outbreak

An unusual outbreak of salmonella infection occurred one September when 49 residents in two small adjoining towns suffered from diarrhoea and vomiting after eating portions of a large 6·35 kg (14 lb) cooked ham from a tin container. The time between ingestion and onset of symptoms varied from 4 to 5 hours, and an unusual member of the salmonella group was isolated from the actual substance of the remainder of the ham, from portions of ham recovered from purchasers, and from stools of all those who suffered from gastroenteritis.

The ham, part of a large consignment of 240 cans received from the Continent, had been preserved with salts in the usual way and pasteurized. This light heat treatment was intended, not to sterilize, but to reduce the bacterial content and to produce an appetizing product. Although sealed in a can for transport purposes, such hams cannot be compared with most canned foods which are given sufficient heat under pressure to kill all bacteria including those which are heat resistant; such sterile packs withstand storage for several years under atmospheric conditions. The manufacturers of 'pasteurized' hams do not intend the packs to be regarded as sterile, for they are usually marked '*Keep in a cool place*', and sometimes '*Perishable—Keep under refrigeration*'.

It is reasonable to suppose that the ham in question was already infected or became contaminated during preparation for packing— in fact before it was cooked—and that subsequent heat treatment failed to kill the contaminants, although leakage into the can of polluted cooking water is another possibility. The bacteriological examination of many samples of ham from pasteurized packs has shown the presence of numerous bacteria of various types. If conditions of storage are poor and the cans are stored in warm, atmospheric temperatures, many become blown and spoiled.

Outbreaks from egg products

For many years outbreaks of salmonellosis and of enteric fever due to *Salmonella paratyphi B* were traced to cream cakes. It was thought that the infection was associated with imitation cream contaminated from human excreters and it took a long time to discover that the source of the contamination was imported bulked egg products; the same types of salmonellae were found in frozen whole egg mixes and in stools from patients suffering from gastro-enteritis and enteric fever. The same phage types of paratyphoid bacilli were persistently found in shipments of cans of frozen egg from China and in the stools of sick patients who had consumed imitation cream products from bakeries using these imported consignments of frozen whole egg.

The imitation cream arrived from the manufacturer in cans and in excellent condition; accidental contamination of the cream with small numbers of salmonellae from egg products occurred in the bakery and conditions for growth were good when the cream was in cakes, éclairs or buns. The egg mixes were rarely if ever a constituent of the cream but mixing bowls, surfaces, utensils and hands served to transfer contamination.

Early in 1963 there were several outbreaks of paratyphoid fever, giving rise to 400 to 500 cases. Cream products from bakeries using

Chinese whole egg were vehicles of infection in all outbreaks and the same types of paratyphoid bacilli causing the illness were isolated from shipments of the frozen whole egg. Legislation to safeguard the product by pasteurization was introduced in 1964 (Chapter 16).

The use of crystalline or pan-dried albumen heavily contaminated with salmonellae has also caused hundreds of cases of salmonellosis. In one outbreak several symptomless excreters of salmonellae who were working in the same bakery and shop were undoubtedly infected from the same source. They in turn were liable to pass on infection by contaminating the foods they handled. Contaminated powdered products may be even more dangerous than liquids from airborne spread and settling in dust on ledges and beams. In Canada there have been serious outbreaks and deaths in children due to the inclusion of contaminated dried egg in prepared cake mixes. In the United States of America contaminated whole egg used uncooked for special diets in hospitals has caused outbreaks. One December, non-acid mayonnaise prepared with contaminated egg mix made many people sick.

Ducks' eggs infected with salmonellae sometimes cause illness, although it is rare now for such incidents to occur. It is worthwhile to relate two outbreaks caused by salmonellae in dishes made with ducks' eggs.

The Queen's pudding outbreak

At least 136 hospital nurses, domestic staff and patients were ill with acute food-poisoning symptoms 24 to 96 hours after they had eaten a particularly appetizing pudding in which the chief ingredients were egg yolk and milk. The yolks of 200 ducks' eggs were beaten with milk and added to breadcrumbs; the mixture was baked for 35 minutes, when it became semi-solid. The top was smeared with hot jam, covered with a layer of beaten-up white of egg mixed with a boiled saturated solution of sugar, and the pudding was returned to the oven for the top to be browned. All those who ate the pudding became ill, including the family of a member of the kitchen staff who had taken some home.

It was generally agreed that the source of infection was contaminated ducks' eggs and that the temperature used to cook the pudding had not been sufficient to kill the bacteria, which could have been present in both the mixtures, one containing yolk and the other egg white. The eggs had been collected from sixteen Essex farms, and

the task of detecting the particular ducks responsible for the contaminated eggs was not practicable. Furthermore, to destroy the
duck population of sixteen farms would have entailed an economic
loss seemingly out of proportion to the chance occurrence of
another food-poisoning outbreak on the same large scale.

The warning to cook all ducks' eggs thoroughly, for at least 10
minutes if they are boiled, and both sides if fried, or better still to
use them only for well-cooked foodstuffs such as baked fruit cakes
or steamed puddings, is frequently given. Lightly baked puddings,
meringues or other foods which may require little or no cooking
should never be made with ducks' eggs for they constitute a
potential danger to the consumer, particularly the very young, the
aged and the invalid. The hazard of cross-contamination from
cake mix made with ducks' eggs to uncooked cream fillings
prepared with the same equipment should also be avoided.

The mousse outbreak (Fig. 14)

The uncooked food vehicle, mousse, prepared with ducks' eggs,
was responsible for salmonellosis in a boys' school. The eggs came
from ducks that lived on a pond near the school, and the sweet was
prepared the day before required.

The cooks placed the mousse overnight in a cool basement room
and the following morning they tasted it before they left for a day's
outing. Unfortunately, in case the sweet should be forgotten, they
removed it from the cool cellar to the warm kitchen where it
remained until eaten by the staff only at the evening meal. The
cooks were apparently unaffected, but next day all the staff were ill
and the boys remained healthy and boisterous. Once again the
lesson was learnt that ducks' eggs should not be used for uncooked
foods and that in any case foods suitable for bacterial growth
should not be kept unrefrigerated.

Coconut

Typhoid fever and salmonellosis were caused by contaminated
desiccated coconut in Australia in 1953. The vehicle was coconut
ball confectionery. Almost as soon as it was known that salmonellae
and paratyphoid bacilli were present in desiccated coconut imported into the United Kingdom, there were reports of cases of
paratyphoid fever and salmonellosis after eating coconut marshmallow biscuits and uncooked coconut. Some foods garnished with

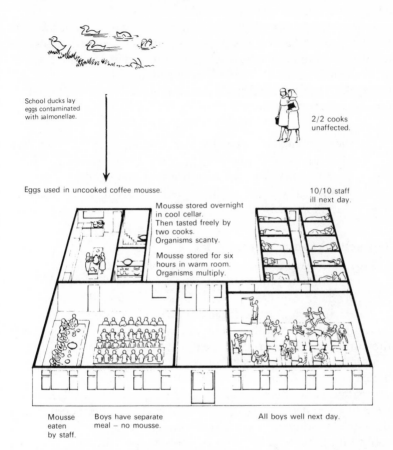

School ducks lay eggs contaminated with salmonellae.

2/2 cooks unaffected.

Eggs used in uncooked coffee mousse.

10/10 staff ill next day.

Mousse stored overnight in cool cellar. Then tasted freely by two cooks. Organisms scanty.

Mousse stored for six hours in warm room. Organisms multiply.

Mousse eaten by staff.

Boys have separate meal – no mousse.

All boys well next day.

FIG. 14. The mousse outbreak. (Mousse: light dish made of beaten white of eggs, etc.)

LABORATORY FINDINGS

S. typhimurium from ducks (cloacal swabs), from ducks' eggs and from faeces of patients.

COMMENTS

1. Ducks' eggs must not be used in uncooked or lightly cooked dishes. They may be used with safety in baked or other well-cooked food, or hard boiled (15 minutes).
2. Foodstuffs prepared some hours before consumption should be stored in the cold.

coconut were able to support and encourage the growth of salmonellae.

Improved conditions of production enforced by legislation in Ceylon brought about a steady drop in the proportion of contaminated samples and suspected incidents. The steam treatment of desiccated coconut to be used uncooked in or on food, which was undertaken voluntarily by many manufacturers, helped to reduce infection from this source.

Another well defined type of food poisoning arises from the contamination, predominantly of meat and poultry dishes, with large numbers of the anaerobic sporing bacillus, *Clostridium welchii*. The following incidents illustrate the sequence of events which can lead to *Cl. welchii* food poisoning.

The school canteen outbreaks

Two outbreaks of food poisoning occurred in the same school canteen within a year of each other. On the first occasion the medical officer of health reported the occurrence of abdominal pain and diarrhoea among a large number of children in a school served by its own canteen. The kitchen was visited the day after the outbreak. The suspected meal, eaten 9 to 12 hours before the symptoms started, consisted of cold boiled salt beef, salad and boiled potatoes, followed by a steamed pudding and jam. The food was eaten without complaint and tasted good. The beef, in joints weighing about 1·8 to 2·7 kg (4 to 6 lb) each, had been delivered to the kitchen on the previous afternoon. The meat was immediately cooked for 2 hours in large boilers of the type commonly found in modern school canteens, and it was allowed to remain in the liquor all night to cool. The following day the meat was taken from the liquor, drained, sliced and eaten cold for lunch. A portion of this meat, left over from the meal and stored in the refrigerator, was examined at the laboratory. Several types of bacteria were found, including the sporing bacillus, *Cl. welchii*. It was assumed that either the spores had survived the preliminary heat treatment or that airborne contamination had occurred during cooling, and that multiplication had been vigorous overnight. The kitchen staff were warned that the procedure they had used—that of boiling the meat the day before it was required and allowing it to cool slowly overnight in the kitchen—was the most likely explanation for the outbreak. The staff appeared to understand, and agreed that it should not occur again.

Almost exactly a year later, the medical officer of health reported a similar occurrence in the same school, affecting about 200 children. In the meantime, laboratory experiments had proved that the spores of *Cl. welchii*, isolated from many samples of meatstuffs suspected of causing outbreaks of diarrhoea and pain, were able to withstand a few minutes' to several hours' boiling and the story told was similar to that of many other such incidents already reported. For the greater part of the year following the warning given after the first outbreak, the staff had been careful to carry out the recommendation to cook and eat their meat on the same day; occasionally they had refrigerated overnight any meat cooked the day before it was required for a cold meal. For the past few months, however, they had lapsed into their old habits. On this occasion, rolled joints of salt beef had been boiled during the afternoon of the day before they were required. They were lifted out of the boiler on to enamel dishes, covered with cloths, and placed in the larder overnight. They were sliced and eaten cold for lunch the next day. In spite of the fact that it was mid-winter, the cooling rate inside the rolls of meat must have been very much slower than the outside and an almost pure culture of heat-resistant *Cl. welchii* was found in the sample of meat examined. A similar organism was isolated from the faeces of patients (Fig. 15).

These sporing bacilli were most probably on the meat when it reached the canteen; but if the organisms had not been given the opportunity to multiply after cooking by long slow cooling and storage at atmospheric temperature, without refrigeration, food poisoning would have been prevented.

Outbreaks of *Cl. welchii* food poisoning continue to occur; they follow a similar pattern. Sometimes the precooked meat or poultry is eaten cold and sometimes it is warmed up.

Soups, stews and gravies cooked in bulk and allowed to cool slowly may also encourage sporing organisms to multiply to dangerous levels. For example, gravy prepared in bulk at a central school-meals kitchen was distributed to neighbouring schools, after it had stood in a large container in the refrigerator overnight. Several outbreaks of food poisoning occurred among children in the various schools, and the gravy was found to be heavily contaminated with sporing organisms. The amount of fluid contained in the single bowl was large and even after refrigeration overnight the temperature in the centre of the mass was such that the multiplication of micro-organisms could still occur.

In a series of hospital outbreaks it was found that boiled chickens in liquor were transferred to open vessels and left all night to cool; illness followed their consumption cold the following day. On the

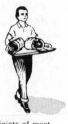

Large joints of meat arrived on Tuesday.

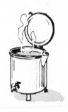

They were boiled on Tuesday afternoon.

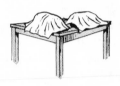

There was no room in the refrigerator, so they were allowed to cool slowly overnight.

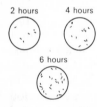

2 hours   4 hours

6 hours

During the night the heat-resistant sporing bacteria grew and multiplied.

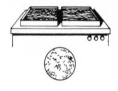

The bacteria multiplied still more when the sliced meat was warmed with gravy on the hot plate.

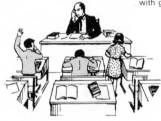

300 ILL

With pain and diarrhoea after 350 children and staff had eaten meat boiled the previous day.

FIG. 15.   Outbreak of *Clostridium welchii* food poisoning in a school canteen

COMMENTS

Meat for hot dishes should be prepared, cooked and eaten the same day. When required cold, cooked meat should be cooled quickly and refrigerated. Joints should be limited to 2·72 kg (6 lb) or less.

other hand, chickens which were removed from the liquor, placed on trays and encouraged to cool quickly, and fed to special-diet patients did not cause illness. *Cl. welchii* was found in a high proportion of dust samples from the kitchen. The organism may have been on the chickens before cooking, it may have been on the containers used for the cooked chickens, or there may have been airborne contamination. Whatever the source, the main fault was the long slow cooling which encouraged multiplication. Figure 16 shows the meats and meat dishes which have caused *Cl. welchii* food poisoning most frequently. There was a marked increase in the incidents of *Cl. welchii* food poisoning in 1963 but the figure dropped again the following year; every year there are appreciable numbers of outbreaks in hospitals and schools.

The curry outbreaks

Near and Far Eastern countries specialize in curries which present a constant hazard of *Cl. welchii* food poisoning. An account of a picnic will illustrate the sequence of events.

The coach started for the Bakra Dam in the Punjab, India, at 7.30 a.m. but the chicken curry had been cooked during the night and it was observed to be present in the coach near the engine, in a large covered metal pan. The day was hot and the journey long. At 2 p.m. the party of 50 persons settled on the grass near the Dam for lunch. The pan of curry was warmed for 10 minutes on a kerosene stove and everyone had generous helpings of curry and rice, which were delicious.

Many hours later 3 people were obviously unwell in the coach, and early the following morning nearly everyone suffered with abdominal pain and diarrhoea. Some of the spores of *Cl. welchii* in poultry and in the spices would survive cooking by boiling and the conditions were ideal for growth and multiplication.

In spite of the warning a similar trip took place the following year with the same menu and the same results. Since no one was sick after 2 hours it is assumed that *Bacillus cereus* was not growing in the rice (see p. 101), although this was another hazard.

Salmonellosis from veal and other meat

The role of animal excreters in human salmonellosis is illustrated by an outbreak of food poisoning involving at least 90 persons in 55 separate incidents. The special typing technique (phage-typing) of the *S. typhimurium* showed that supposed unrelated cases were all part of the same outbreak and that sick calves from a farm many miles away were also infected with the same organism. Calves from this and other farms in the same area were slaughtered in abattoirs providing meat for shops in the districts affected by food

CL. WELCHII PRODUCING HEAT-RESISTANT SPORES
IS A COMMON CONTAMINANT OF MEAT AND POULTRY.

STEWING STEAK
precooked for pies
and pasties.
Heated later to
cook pastry only.

LEG OF MUTTON
for boiling.

ROLLED BRISKET
for boiling or roasting.

CHICKEN
for boiling.

Precooked some hours before required.

COMMON FAULTS IN COOKING, STORAGE AND HANDLING TECHNIQUES
ALLOW SURVIVAL OF SPORES AND MULTIPLICATION OF BACILLI.

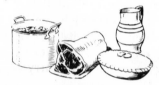 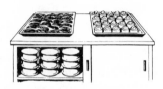

STEWS, STOCK, GRAVY
AND LARGE CUTS OF MEAT
allowed to cool slowly and
stored at room temperature.

SLICED MEAT IN GRAVY
AND 'VOL-AU-VENT'
kept warm for 2 hours or more
on hot plate at about 35°–48°C.

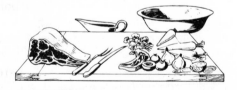

SPORES transferred from raw to cooked meat during boning and slicing
by common surfaces and utensils. The human carrier may also play a part.

FIG. 16. *Clostridium welchii* food poisoning—from meats

COMMENTS
Meat dishes should be freshly prepared and eaten hot within 1 hour of cooking or cooled rapidly and refrigerated until required. Spores can be killed by pressure cooking and the thorough roasting of small cuts of meat.

poisoning. Calf meat in one form or another was the probable vehicle of infection.

The examination of faecal samples taken at farms from more than a thousand calves showed that approximately 0·5 per cent of the faeces of the animals were infected. However, when faecal samples were taken from calves from the same areas, but after the animals had been herded together in collecting centres for 2 to 5 days under poor conditions, 36 per cent of faecal samples were positive for salmonellae and a high proportion gave the epidemic type. Thus stress and cross-infection were important factors.

Many outbreaks with a similar history have been related to pork products made from carcasses contaminated by salmonellae from the intestinal contents of the pig. Ham, sausages, faggots and pork joints have all been implicated in outbreaks of salmonellosis, and in some instances the same types of salmonellae have been isolated from the living animals, the environment of the slaughterhouse and carcasses, glands and offal.

Sometimes sick animals inadvertently killed in the abattoir have led to a heavy contamination of the environment; sometimes the animals have been kept many days before slaughter so that infection from a few has spread to many, encouraged by poor conditions. A similar situation arises with poultry and poultry meat.

The most likely single source of infection is the feeding stuffs, such as bone, fish and meat meals fed to the animals on the farm. The numbers of salmonellae in the meals are usually small so that the animals remain well, but some retain the organism. The rate of excretion on the farm is low because the animals are living under normal conditions but when the creatures are exposed to stress by travel, unfamiliar weather conditions, overcrowding and fighting the rate of excretion rises and the infection spreads.

The amount of general contamination arising because of these factors will vary according to the level of hygiene in the establishments concerned, but these hazards cannot all be removed until feeding stuffs for animals are themselves freed from salmonellae (Fig. 17).

Salmonella outbreaks

The role of infected poultry and animals in the spread of salmonellae to carcass meat and so to the human population is illustrated by four out of many outbreaks of food poisoning.

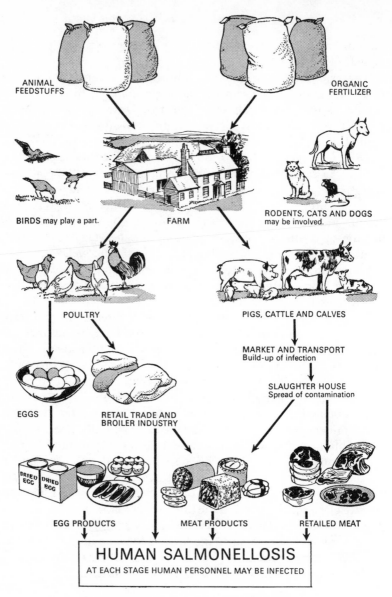

ANIMAL FEEDSTUFFS

ORGANIC FERTILIZER

BIRDS may play a part.

FARM

RODENTS, CATS AND DOGS may be involved.

POULTRY

PIGS, CATTLE AND CALVES

MARKET AND TRANSPORT
Build-up of infection

SLAUGHTER HOUSE
Spread of contamination

EGGS

RETAIL TRADE AND BROILER INDUSTRY

DRIED EGG   DRIED EGG

EGG PRODUCTS

MEAT PRODUCTS

RETAILED MEAT

HUMAN SALMONELLOSIS
AT EACH STAGE HUMAN PERSONNEL MAY BE INFECTED

Fig. 17.   Spread of salmonella contamination

PREVENTIVE MEASURES INCLUDE:

1. Improved hygiene of production in country of origin, on farms, in markets, slaughterhouses and in factories.
2. Treatment of foods liable to contamination including human and animal foodstuffs by pasteurization, dry heat, irradiation and other methods.

Salmonella virchow

Several episodes of salmonella food poisoning, four of which involved at least 140 people, were reported in 1968. They were all associated with chicken meals and spit-roasting was a prominent feature of cooking methods.

Some investigators thought that the organism survived in the cooked birds because they were not completely thawed before cooking which may have been too rapid. Others thought that salmonellae were transferred from the raw debris left on surfaces, utensils, cloths and hands to cooked birds after removal from the spit and during subsequent cutting-up operations. The source of the infection of the dressed poultry was live birds which are likely to have picked up infection from feed meals. The next fault was storage after cooking. Warm spit-roasted carcasses pending sale will encourage multiplication of a scanty contamination; likewise non-chilled storage in the kitchen will encourage growth. Food-handlers, victims of the foods they handle, were found to be excreting *S. virchow* but the part played by their faecal excretion would be minimal or non-existent compared with their part in the mechanical spread by hands and utensils from the masses of infected raw birds to the cooked product.

Salmonella senftenberg

For many years a small hospital was invaded by this salmonella serotype. At one stage a third of the hospital staff were excreting *S. senftenberg* and the number of sick people increased. The hospital was closed temporarily, thus disrupting the work and the training of nurses. Many excreters were found in the kitchen as well as amongst patients, nurses and doctors. It was noteworthy that the staff of two departments who ate food prepared at home and not in the canteen were not found to be excreters.

Turkeys were a fairly regular feature of the diet and they came from an area some distance away, where outbreaks of salmonellosis due to *S. senftenberg* had occurred amongst the flocks. Long and arduous tracking eventually established that turkeys from infected farms were supplied to the hospital. Other hospitals were supplied also but the method of cooking was particularly light in the hospital concerned, and there were environmental faults which would have encouraged the spread of salmonellae in the kitchen. An additional factor was the proximity of a pig farm to windward of the prefabricated kitchen building. The farmer mixed his own feed and the ingredients would be contaminated with *S. senftenberg* from time to time.

Salmonella typhimurium phage type 32

A widespread outbreak of salmonellosis from *S. typhimurium* phage type 32 resulted in hundreds of cases of food poisoning and 12 deaths in a Scottish city. Pork meat products from many shops all over the city were vehicles of infection and the same strain was isolated from live pigs in the large local abattoir and also from the gut room and drains. *S. typhimurium* phage type 32 was also found in 4 of 10 samples of a feeding stuff ingredient produced locally for various farms. It was never fully established whether this phage type was recirculated in feeding stuffs compounded from rendered lots of infected pork or whether it had suddenly appeared from an imported ingredient. The outbreak died down, so presumably the focus of infection disappeared.

During the height of the outbreak cases occurred in England, in an area receiving pork carcasses from the Scottish abattoir. Of two hospitals, both receiving the same pork meat, one, with a bad kitchen, reported cases of salmonellosis due to the same organism. The other, with a good kitchen, remained free from cases. In the bad kitchen, lighting, surfaces, utensils and general morale were poor; the good kitchen was a model of lightness, new equipment, cleanliness and efficiency.

Salmonella brandenburg

The incidence of human cases and symptomless excreters of *S. brandenburg* increased 37 times during a period of 5 years and 18 times during a period of 1 year. Over the same period of time *S. brandenburg* was found in 12 per cent of samples of minced meat prepared for sausages by two factories. The organism was found in 12 of 24 pens in the relevant abattoir where pigs were kept for 2 days to 1 month or longer (now illegal) before slaughter. Sewer swabs were also positive. When appropriate measures were taken there were improvements in the isolation rates of the *S. brandenburg* in factory products and the abattoir and the incidence of food poisoning due to this organism dropped. Although it proved impossible to track the organism back to its source, it was assumed that one or more farms were responsible for the infected pigs. *S. brandenburg* has been isolated many times from imported meat and bone meal.

The contaminated pies outbreak

It is probable that outbreaks of salmonella food poisoning from meat pies are caused usually by contaminated meat supplies and that symptomless excreters among food handlers are victims rather than originators of infection. An outbreak from meat pies which occurred in July 1949 is described. 206 pies and 450 sausage rolls were made by a Midland firm and distributed to twelve branches. Of those who ate the pies, 29 of 11 family groups and 21 Scouts at camp in Scotland became acutely ill with food-poisoning symptoms 5 to 24 hours later, while those who ate the sausage rolls were unaffected. A dog fed with the remains of a pie which gave rise to human cases likewise suffered from acute gastroenteritis. Twenty-one of the 27 members of the Scout camp were taken ill their first night in camp. Rain which started heavily that night continued for 6 days; the latrine had been dug in a distant part of the field. For nearly 3 weeks the camp was never free of invalids; some developed high temperatures and were transferred to the local hospital and houses in the district. In 2 cases recovery was not complete until October. Organisms of the salmonella group were isolated from the stools of patients, from a symptomless excreter and from 13 meat pies. There were both large and small pies, but the attack rate was higher among those who ate the large pies on the first day after manufacture, although by the second day the small pies were causing severe diarrhoea and the severity of illness varied with the quantity of pie eaten.

The bakery at which the pies had been made employed about 100 persons; their standard of cleanliness was high and there was good sanitary accommodation. The same consignment of meat had been used for both pies and sausage rolls; it had been minced, seasoned and mixed with 'filler'. The prepared meat was hand-filled into the pastry blocks by three persons. The pies were heated for 25 to 30 minutes at 232 to 246°C (450 to 475°F) and the gelatin was added after baking; sheet gelatin was soaked in water, dissolved in fresh boiling water, and cooled and filled into the pies from a jug. The pies were stored at room temperature overnight and distributed next day. It seemed that the cooking time and temperature were adequate to sterilize the sausage rolls but not the pies. The higher attack rate from the large pies eaten on the first day of manufacture indicates that the heat penetration into these pies was slower than for the small size and that therefore more bacteria survived the cooking in the large pies.

An examination of stool samples showed that one of the three pie makers was excreting salmonella organisms. She was probably a victim through eating raw pie meat as was her custom. Specimens of sheet gelatin, washings from the tin used for the gelatin, a mouse trapped in the bakery, and specimens from six batches of pies prepared subsequently were examined bacteriologically with negative results.

Conditions in the butcher's shop from which the meat was obtained were far from satisfactory, but the most likely source of the organism was the carcass meat used for the mince.

Food-poisoning outbreaks due to meat pies occur from time to time. It seems that they will continue to do so until steps are taken to ensure that the times and temperatures of cooking are such that the raw meat is well cooked, even though the pastry may become over-brown in consequence. The use of precooked meat in pies is not a safe alternative. Heat-resistant spores may survive the first cooking and develop into actively growing bacilli in meat left overnight; the new growth of organisms may not be destroyed by the cooking time and temperature needed merely to bake the pastry and warm through the meat. Great care should also be taken with the gelatin which is poured into the pie after it is cooked. It should be boiled and filled into the pies hot, not less than 65·6 °C (150 °F); the pies should then be cooled rapidly and maintained in the cold until required.

Salmonellae may be found in a small proportion of home-killed meat on sale in butchers' shops, and in a much larger percentage of frozen boneless meat, for both human and animal consumption (see Chapter 4, Table 8). Boneless packs of veal, beef and mutton are used by manufacturers for pies and sausages as well as for canning. It is not surprising therefore that samples of un-cooked sausages and minced meat contain salmonellae. The proportion of samples found to be positive will depend on the raw meat itself.

Milk

Salmonella and staphylococcal outbreaks from unpasteurized milk are not uncommon. In staphylococcal outbreaks the cow's udder excretes staphylococci into the milk. Salmonellae may come from the faeces or even from the udder of the cow; polluted water, feeding stuffs, other livestock and human excreters may be involved.

The following description of an outbreak illustrates the paths of spread of infection, when 58 of 900 people including children were infected by raw TT milk contaminated with *S. typhimurium* during October and November, 1960. The dairy, run by the owner and one employee, sold 227 to 273 litres (50 to 60 gallons) per day of raw TT milk bottled on the premises but purchased from a farm nearby. The dairyman and his family lived on the premises, the employee elsewhere. Near the house the dairyman kept several hundred hens in deep litter houses.

The farmer concerned milked about 40 cattle. One cow was clinically suspect, another had been sold to the knacker's yard, and the farmer had suffered from diarrhoea a fortnight earlier. *S. typhimurium* was isolated from a milk sample taken from the dairy, from stools from three of the dairyman's family and his employee, from three members of the farmer's family and from two rectal swabs taken from the cattle—one from the sick beast. All the strains of *S. typhimurium* were of the same phage type. The milk samples from the farm were negative, and so was the water. It was assumed that the milk was contaminated in the cowshed, the milk-room, or in the bottling plant of the dairy. Cowshed dung could have been responsible and in the milk-room contamination could have been introduced by vessels or by hands contaminated by the cows. Milk at the dairy could have been infected in the bottling plant by the positive dairyman's assistant but it was suspected that the infection originated from the farm, possibly from the farmer himself. Wet weather may have helped to spread infection because the tails, legs and udders of the cattle were dirty. Other possible sources of infection were hens and grazing land.

Formal notice was served requiring heat treatment of the milk. It is stressed that no milk is safe unless pasteurized. The sale of raw milk in vending machines and for schools should be strictly forbidden.

The rice outbreak

Fried rice with high counts of *Bacillus cereus* have been responsible for acute vomiting, sometimes followed by diarrhoea, in people eating food prepared in Chinese restaurants. The rapid onset of sickness usually within 2–4 hours of eating the food suggests that a toxin is released in the food. *B. cereus* spores readily and grows well at a wide range of temperatures. The spores can withstand near-boiling temperatures, particularly when protected by starch. In order to be ready to provide take-away meals at a moment's notice, large quantities of rice may be boiled the day before required and sometimes they are piled high in large colanders and left overnight in the kitchen. Refrigeration is said to coagulate the particles. Portions are turned over in hot fat (fried) in the morning and kept warm pending sale, when they are flipped through hot fat in a final process.

The nature of the organisms suggests that the spores are present in the dried rice, survive boiling and germinate into bacilli which grow rapidly in the cooked rice. The spores are formed quickly in most vegetative cells so that the second process of heating in oil still leaves spores alive to germinate and form more sporing cells which are not disturbed by the final treatment in hot fat. The effect of heat on the toxin is not known but it is possible that it withstands some of the cooking procedure.

Only a revision in the method of preparation to cut out the hours of storage between and after cooking will prevent this type of food poisoning.

Vibrio parahaemolyticus from the East

Passengers travelling by air from Bangkok via Dubai were taken ill as they arrived in London. Three who reported sick immediately were taken to hospital; information about other cases came later. Aircrew who landed at Dubai and did not proceed to London were also ill; this established the food vehicles as part of a meal prepared in Bangkok and eaten before the aircraft reached Dubai. Crab hors d'œuvre was suspected. All foods were examined but *V. parahaemolyticus*, isolated from the cooked crab meat, was the organism also isolated from stool samples of the three hospitalized patients. Raw meat from crab claws flown from Bangkok also harboured *V. parahaemolyticus*.

There were two possibilities: either the organism was not killed in the process of boiling, or the cooked crab meat was recontaminated with the organism from the raw meat during extraction from the shell and preparation and assembly of the crab and sweet corn salad. When an organism has been once recognized as a potential cause of trouble in food it can be found more readily the next time. The isolation of *V. parahaemolyticus* from imported frozen cooked prawns suggests the possibility of sickness from prawn cocktails.

The contamination of cooked crab by *V. parahaemolyticus* in uncooked crabs during picnics has been described in the USA outbreaks.

V. parahaemolyticus food poisoning has been described frequently in the East but air travel and imported foods bring East to West with rapidity. The same is true for cholera but built-in safeguards for sewage and water control will protect the West, at least from widespread water-borne outbreaks of infection.

7
Ecology of Micro-organisms in Food

As regular co-inhabitants of this world, micro-organisms must not only survive but also multiply actively so that replacements are available for the frequent losses of microbial population. The spoilage organisms have less difficulty in maintaining their existence than those which depend on occupation of the human or animal body. They proliferate readily in almost any protein material or vegetable matter at a wide range of ambient temperatures. The pathogens, on the other hand, depend on the warmth and nutriment of the animal and human body for growth; if they conquer then life dies with the host and they must seek another foothold in other susceptible hosts. At an intermediate stage foods are useful for growth when temperatures are suitable, or, when they are unsuitable, for resting phases. The characteristics of organisms in relation to the food and the living habitat, and also to survival outside both, can be the subject of an ecological study for each type or organism. Broad patterns of behaviour can be seen within the families which include the clostridia, staphylococci, salmonellae and dysentery bacilli, aerobic sporing bacilli such as *Bacillus cereus* and the vibrios.

Clostridium

Consider the genus *Clostridium* and in particular *Clostridium welchii*. This organism flourishes under anaerobic conditions in the lower intestinal tract and in deep wounds. In the large bowel of man and animals it spores readily and the spores will pass out with the faeces into soil or sewage systems. Water and vegetation will carry it back into the animal kingdom and into food production systems including kitchens, where it arrives in meats, vegetables and dust. The mechanism of heat resistance enables the spores to survive normal cooking procedures. The heat of cooking activates the spores to germinate, possibly by damaging the spore coat.

When the slowly cooling foods (usually meat and poultry) reach the satisfactory temperature for growth (below 50 °C; 122 °F) there

104

is rapid multiplication of the vegetative cells emerging from the spores; swallowed with food they must survive the acid conditions of the stomach and reach the intestine in sufficient numbers. Once more inside the human or animal body they disturb the natural flora so that conditions are right for multiplication and sporulation to take place. A particularly large dose must be present in the food for the phenomenon known as diarrhoea, accompanied by cramps, to occur. Large numbers of cells and spores will be excreted in the large volume of fluid stool until the normal flora is restored.

The spores can survive indefinitely and they are resistant to environmental factors such as dehydration, heat and cold. Another characteristic of this organism is its fast generation time under congenial conditions. Divisions occur every 10 to 12 minutes at a wide range of temperatures, the optimum being 43 to 47 °C (109·4 to 116·6 °F); the maximum temperature is about 50 °C (122 °F) and the minimum about 20 °C. The mode of attack is not from toxin formed in the food but from toxin released in the intestine, it is suggested as a result of sporulation. The organism is known to produce large numbers of spores in the intestine but not in the foodstuffs. The outflow of spores as well as vegetative cells from those suffering from food poisoning will be profuse and contribute to the survival and spread of the organism. The other more lethal organism of the same family, *Cl. botulinum*, forms its toxin when growing in the food. It has been suggested only recently that there may be growth and toxin production within wounds, and in the intestine of poultry infected by *Cl. botulinum* type C in the disease called limberneck.

The toxin which causes the fatal nerve disease of botulism is formed in food and fortunately it is sensitive to heat otherwise there would be more fatalities in those eating cooked foods. The general incidence of the organism *Cl. botulinum* in soil and food appears to be low, and it has been found only in certain areas. There are no records of the number of *Cl. botulinum* in the stools of the victims. The gastrointestinal phase of the illness is transient and suspected to be due to organisms other than *Cl. botulinum* in the same food. The sparse incidence of the organism may be associated with the rarity of the disease compared with *Cl. welchii* food poisoning and with the fact that it is not excreted profusely in the stool, in contrast to *Cl. welchii*. It has been suggested that the main natural source of *Cl. botulinum* type C, an animal pathogen, is the carcasses of dead animals and maybe the alimentary tract of live animals.

Multiplication in excreted faecal material has also been suggested. The cycle for spread and survival of *Cl. botulinum* type E in fish, coastal mud and water may be the same, with man and his sewage as a contributory factor. The victim of botulism often dies as a result of the toxin which may influence the survival of the organism outside the human and animal host. Perhaps the cycle can be perpetuated with small doses of the organism in food although the system will be inefficient without the onset of clinical symptoms.

Staphylococcus

It is doubtful whether the staphylococci have an intermediate environmental phase of significance unless it be dust. Their perpetuation is not dependent on faecal excretion; it is assured in the warm damp and congenial atmosphere of the nose and throat, in the pores and hair follicles of the skin and on the surface of skin in damp creased areas such as the perineum and axillae. It is not easy to rid the skin, or the nose, of staphylococci of any type. Measures have been suggested such as antibiotic creams for the nose; these at least can eliminate a particular type which may be giving rise to skin lesions or known to produce enterotoxin in food. Freedom from the organism may be transient but the next invader may be less harmful.

Bactericidal soaps and lotions for the skin are described but they require persistent and consistent usage to be effective. Washing the skin with soap and water usually eliminates gram-negative bacilli, but gram-positive cocci often remain and sometimes appear in even greater numbers. They rise to the surface of the skin from pores when the hands are soaked or rinsed in hot water; superficial layers of the skin are disturbed by scrubbing and rubbing which may even distribute the organisms over the surface.

If a moist cake of soap is passed gently over the surface of agar medium in a petri dish, organisms common to the skin of whoever is using the soap will be demonstrated by colonies growing on the plate after incubation.

Breaks in the skin surface will encourage proliferation, and septic lesions forming pus will release enormous numbers of cells which may linger on the skin indefinitely. Growth in food is a poor means of perpetuation. The enterotoxins which cause illness are produced in the food and the number of cells excreted in the faeces at the time of illness or at any other time does not appear to be great. This will not be true for another condition giving rise to staphylococcal enteritis which sometimes follows administration of antibiotics disturbing the natural flora of the intestine. Staphylococci may then become dominant and be excreted in large numbers; but, unlike the sporing organisms, the time of survival of the vegetative cells outside the body will be limited.

Compared with the gram-negative and positive bacilli, staphylococci are slow in competitive growth and they need the body temperature to proliferate; thus the organism is dependent on living tissue. There is a high incidence of staphylococci (including *Staph. aureus*) on live poultry and on the skin of dressed poultry but the types are rarely associated with food poisoning. Investigations have been carried out on enterotoxins produced by strains of staphylococci isolated in large numbers from foods associated with food poisoning, and those isolated in small numbers during the routine examination of various foods. The results show a close association between the food-poisoning strain and those frequently isolated from man and known to produce enterotoxin, and a low correlation between strains known to produce enterotoxin and those found during the routine examination of foods, not associated with food poisoning.

Phage typing has enabled the spread of staphylococci to be followed more closely, and is a useful epidemiological tool.

Salmonella

The ramifications of the various organisms of the salmonella group are far and wide, the ecology is complex and the damage to animals as well as to man is immense.

Perhaps because the natural course of events is the surest means of survival, the salmonella cycle is predominantly in countries where there are vast schemes for the intensive rearing of animals. The waste products and remains of animals, whether sick or healthy are not carefully channelled into safe sewage disposal schemes or buried or burned but they are processed into feeding stuffs and fertilizers and placed back in the cycle of infection.

If the methods of processing rendered them sterile or at least free from pathogens which infect both man and animals, the economy of the animal–feed–animal–food–man system would be perfect. But unless special precautions are taken the finished feed products from rendered animal products are frequently contaminated with salmonellae which are fed back to the animals. It has been demonstrated that the number of animals (or poultry) in any group found to be excreting salmonellae is dependent on contamination of the feeding stuffs used in the unit.

The animal intestine is as conducive for the survival and multiplication of samonellae as that of man. The animal system has the added advantage of rapid spread between animals in overcrowded conditions; of the probability of survival and multiplication in rehydrated mash in troughs and lairages where trauma between animals may lead to lowered resistance to infection of the animal body; of anxiety and stress in transport and strange surroundings and, at times, of deprivation of food and water in days before slaughter. All these factors predispose the animal to infection and will enhance excretion.

Except under war conditions and vast antisocial campaigns, humanity is rarely subjected to these circumstances and except for excretion into sewage the invading organisms may live and die with the host only.

The use of antibiotics will be more effective in man since both the type of antibiotic and the dose will be controlled more carefully. However, in animals small doses in feeds or for prophylaxis will perpetuate resistant strains of pathogens and non-pathogens and resistance factors may be active in the transfer mechanism even in the absence of antibiotics. Doses for treatment of scouring animals will, more often than not, be given without knowledge of the organism concerned and therefore of its sensitivity. Statistical records of salmonellosis in animals are mostly made up from post-mortem findings from animals brought into veterinary investigation laboratories.

Comparative studies have been carried out with the Danes. In Denmark dehydrated protein feeding stuffs of animal origin are required to be salmonella-free and there is legislation for heat treatment. Pigs in Denmark have a lower rate of excretion and it is significant that *S. typhimurium* is the predominant serotype in pigs and in the population; whereas in the UK other serotypes are prominent both in animals and man, and many of these are found in foodstuffs both for man and animals. The Danes have a pathogen-free programme for poultry which relates not only to foodstuffs but also to all stages in breeding. The success of this system is shown by the freedom from salmonellae, except for an occasional batch with *S. typhimurium*, of poultry carcasses and pieces imported from Denmark and examined in the United Kingdom.

The effect of allowing animals for domestic consumption to eat salmonellae in their food is reflected in the incidence of the organism in raw products—particularly comminuted meats such as sausages and also dressed poultry. There are wide differences in the rate of contamination of meat and poultry products between enlightened manufacturers and breeders, including those responsible for slaughtering.

A partial reduction in the incidence of salmonellosis may be brought about by efforts to prevent spread of infection from raw to cooked products at the retail-consumer end of the chain; but without international co-operation of the disciplines responsible for animal care, the intestinal disease of salmonellosis will persist.

Bacillus cereus

This is another organism which is troublesome because of its ability to survive indefinitely by means of spores. It may be even more ubiquitous than the sporing clostridia, because it is an aerobic organism not dependent on an oxygen-free environment for growth, and also it forms spores freely; under good conditions for its growth spores are formed in almost every cell. The organism is a common contaminant of cereals and can cause spoilage in cereal-type foods as well as milk and dairy products.

Cornflour sauce, milk puddings and rice dishes have been described as vehicles of infection for man. The survival of the spores through the cooking process, germination, proliferation and production of toxin in food are responsible for human sickness. Harmless though they are in small numbers, the fault lies in the rise of numbers in food prepared in bulk ahead of requirements. Rice for the take-away trade is an example (p. 101).

There is no problem about this organism perpetuating its existence in the world; its control rests with preventing multiplication by allowing short intervals only between cooking and eating, and the full use of refrigeration.

Vibrio parahaemolyticus

The ecology of *V. parahaemolyticus* appears to be closely connected with a water–sea creature cycle; outbreaks, described mostly in Japan, are associated with the consumption of sea food whether raw or cooked. There are no reports of water-borne outbreaks of *V. parahaemolyticus*, unlike those for the cholera vibrio which emphasize the importance of polluted water supplies and sanitary incompetence in the rapid spread of cholera. In eastern countries, for example where cholera is epidemic, *V. parahaemoly-ticus* has also been isolated from stools of persons with cholera-like symptoms when the cholera vibrio itself has not been found.

When sewage becomes overloaded with *V. cholerae* the local water will be invaded by the organism and where there is no purification system the people suffer.

Whereas *V. cholerae* has a second vehicle, food, *V. parahaemolyticus* appears to be dependent on food for transmission through to the human body. This phenomenon may be dependent on the size of the dose, *V. parahaemolyticus* requiring more organisms to cause disease than the cholera vibrio.

In Japan food poisoning due to *V. parahaemolyticus* and the isolation of the organism from coastal waters is a summertime occurrence, and warmth and bacterial growth go hand in hand. Although *V. parahaemolyticus* has been isolated from coastal waters and sea creatures in England, Germany and other countries, the numbers will be small compared with those which accumulate in the environment in epidemic periods in warm Japan; infected sewage from sporadic cases and outbreaks will contribute large numbers of organisms.

Will the sewage from rare incidents such as that described on p. 102 be sufficient to infiltrate the vibrio into water systems and seafoods in other countries? What of the frozen cooked seafoods imported from eastern countries and found to contain *V. para-haemolyticus*? Efficient sewage and water systems will keep most water-borne outbreaks under control but the use or disposal of contaminated imported food is another matter.

8
Food-borne Infection

There are many diseases spread by food which are distinguishable from the acute bacterial food poisoning described in the previous chapters. Some cause illness when small numbers of organisms are swallowed, whereas large numbers of food-poisoning bacteria are required to initiate symptoms. Thus typhoid fever, cholera and dysentery may be water-borne and food is a vehicle of transport for the bacteria passing from source to victim and not necessarily a medium for multiplication.

Paratyphoid fever has two forms, one simulating gastroenteritis and the other enteric fever. The gastroenteritis form has similar symptoms and incubation periods to salmonellosis and is likely to require a fairly large dose of organisms, which means they need time for their multiplication in food. The enteric fever form with symptoms similar to but less severe than typhoid requires 7 to 10 days for incubation, but nothing is known about the dosage. The fact that paratyphoid fever is occasionally water borne suggests that this form may occur after the ingestion of a comparatively small dose of organisms.

Cholera is both water borne and food borne; it spreads rapidly, which indicates secondary infection by person-to-person and environment-to-person spread. The same may also be said for dysentery, though water-borne disease is rare in Great Britain.

Viral agents of food- and water-borne diseases must also be infective in small doses because they cannot multiply in inanimate matter.

The virus of poliomyelitis may be isolated from faeces and sewage; it must be assumed therefore that it can also be food and water borne. The vehicle of infection for the virus of hepatitis, in spite of difficulties in isolation and growth, is thought to include water, shell-fish and food.

It is suspected that other viruses cause gastroenteritis because there are certain outbreaks which cannot be attributed to any of the usual agents, and where the symptoms and incubation periods are compatible with those of virus infection. The difficulty of isolating viruses from faecal and particularly food materials is a hindrance to the investigations.

The incubation period for typhoid fever is 7 to 21 days; it may be less or more according to the dose and the immunity of the individual. The two forms of paratyphoid fever have already been described, the incubation periods being 24 hours or so for the one and 7 to 10 days for the other.

The enteric fevers may begin insidiously with general malaise and fever. Intestinal symptoms may or may not appear early but they are not prominent until the second and third week of fever. The incubation period for dysentery is from 2 to 4 days and acute diarrhoea may persist for several days. The virus diseases usually have long incubation periods of 10 or more days. Gastroenteritis, however, which is often attributed to viruses, may have a short incubation of 1 to 2 days, as shown by groups of people taken ill while attending conferences.

It is convenient to consider the water- and food-borne diseases under the headings, water, milk, ice-cream and food.

Water

After the incident of the Broad Street pump in 1854 when sewage pollution of the district well gave rise to a large-scale outbreak of cholera and many deaths, the famous epidemiologist John Snow turned public attention to water and sanitation. Early in the twentieth century chlorination of mains water was introduced by Alexander Houston. Except for occasional incidents of typhoid fever from well water and small unchlorinated supplies in country districts there was no more trouble until the big Croydon outbreak in 1937. Then 341 persons became ill owing to the introduction into the water supply of typhoid bacilli from the urine of a symptomless excreter working on repairs to a deep well.

In 1963 holiday makers were arriving back from Zermatt and developing typhoid fever, and many Swiss and other holiday makers were ill because sewage had seeped into an undetected leak in the mains water pipe.

There have been instances where adults and children have imbibed contaminated river and stream waters sometimes after falling in accidentally or with suicidal intent and subsequently developed typhoid fever.

In one such instance the origin of *Salmonella typhi* in a stream was traced to symptomless excreters; 11 were found in a mental hospital. The sewage effluent from the hospital discharged into the stream approximately half a mile away from the point near the road where two boys had been playing and drinking the water.

Water may be an indirect source of *S. typhi* when the immediate vehicle is a foodstuff. Shell-fish, oysters for example, may feed and grow in sewage-polluted water. There is a rapid circulation of water through the body of oysters and mussels, during which bacteria, including pathogenic bacteria, are filtered off. The last outbreak traced to this source was in 1958 when oysters from the estuary of the river at West Mersea caused illness. A carrier was excreting *S. typhi* into the river.

Another important and indirect source of *S. typhi* is sewage-polluted river water used for cooling heat-sterilized cans of food. Minute faults in the can structure will allow the water to seep in, particularly as the hot can is under vacuum, so that a few organisms or even one only may be sucked through and contaminate the contents.

S. typhi has been found in a small can of cream; its suspected presence in cans of corned beef and tongue and the resulting outbreaks of typhoid fever are described later in this chapter under Food.

Any pathogenic micro-organism including viruses living in or passing through the intestinal tract of human beings or animals may be transmissible by untreated water polluted by sewage. But the number of organisms required to initiate disease from drinking water must be small unless there is gross pollution. If polluted water is used for purposes of food manufacture then small numbers of pathogenic organisms from water could multiply in the food if conditions were favourable; for example, *S. typhi* growing in canned corned beef and tongue.

Milk

Milk is an ideal medium for bacterial growth and means of contamination are numerous. It may be already dangerously contaminated when taken from the cow. Tuberculous cattle excreting tubercle bacilli in milk used to be one of the main sources of tuberculosis in children and adults. Thirty years ago in Britain there were 4,000 or more new cases of tuberculosis yearly caused by bovine tubercle bacilli. The eradication scheme, including tuberculin testing of cattle and pasteurization of milk, has reduced the incidence almost to vanishing point.

Brucella abortus, the bacillus responsible for abortion in cows, may be excreted in milk and give rise to an infection known as undulant fever in those who consume contaminated raw dairy products such as milk, cream and 'cream' cheese. Farm workers in close proximity to such cattle may also acquire the infection.

Goats and their products may be similarly infected. Undulant fever in man is not often fatal but may cause ill health over long periods of time. Eradication schemes have been successful in Scandinavia and the United States of America.

Infection of the udder, known as mastitis, may lead to excretion of food-poisoning staphylococci, haemolytic streptococci or even salmonellae in the milk. The faeces of the cows infected with salmonellae may contaminate milk directly. In the intimate association between farm workers and their animals diseases are spread from one to the other, and the organisms causing infections in farmers and their helpers may spread to milk. Diphtheria bacilli from human cases and carriers may be implanted on ulcers of the teats of the cows and cause contamination of the milk in this way.

There have been widespread outbreaks of scarlet fever and tonsillitis from streptococci passing into milk from infected lesions in the udder and on the teats of cows. Occasionally, milkers with streptococcal infections have been involved. In one large outbreak pupils in two schools were infected by drinking raw milk. Haemolytic streptococci of the same type were found in the throats of 87 children with scarlet fever, the throats of the milker and his two children, and in the milk. The danger from the spread of infection by those handling cows and milk is lessened by the automatic machine method of milking. Outbreaks of dysentery, typhoid and paratyphoid fever, and of salmonella food poisoning have been spread by milk contaminated by carriers amongst farm and dairy workers but the cow herself is also a likely source of pathogenic organisms. Widespread outbreaks of paratyphoid fever have occurred; more than 1,000 people were infected in one outbreak by drinking raw milk from cows excreting *S. paratyphi B*.

Pails, milking machines and milk bottles may be washed with water polluted with human or animal sewage. Recommended chlorine compounds are available for use on farms, and milk bottles should be rinsed, washed in detergent and rinsed in very hot water followed by cool mains water. Chlorine is sometimes used in rinse waters also.

In spite of all the hygienic precautions which may be taken on farms, bottling depots and dairies, the only method to safeguard

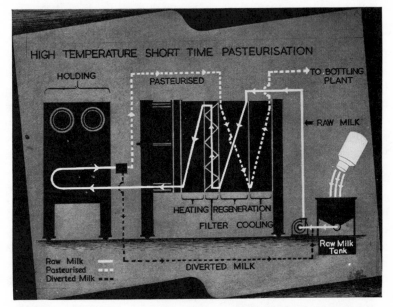

Fig. 18. Diagram of pasteurization plant (High Temperature Short Time method)

milk for delivery to the consumer is by heat treatment before or after it has been bottled and capped. By this means all pathogenic organisms introduced from the cow, from subsequent contacts or other sources will be destroyed and there will be no further danger of contamination until the bottled milk reaches the consumer's kitchen. Here the milk is subject to the hazards of household use, but with reasonable care and cold storage it may be kept safe.

There are two commercial methods for heat treatment: one is by pasteurization, which is usually carried out in a plant as illustrated in Fig. 18, and the other by disinfection at a temperature of 100°C (212°F) or over. The latest method which may in time replace all other methods of heat treatment is by steam infiltration, which necessitates aseptic filling but provides milk with a long shelf life (see Chapter 2, p. 18; Chapter 16, pp. 232–233).

The following description of a typhoid incident illustrates some of the points mentioned.

Typhoid fever from raw milk

An extensive outbreak of milk-borne disease occurred one autumn in the adjacent towns of Christchurch, Poole and Bournemouth. There were 518 cases among the local inhabitants and about 200 persons were infected while on holiday in the district, although the disease did not develop until they returned home; there were about 70 deaths. Men, women and children of all ages and occupation were affected. This suggested infection by a common food of wide distribution; milk was an obvious possibility. It was soon discovered that all the primary cases had consumed raw milk from one particular dairy. Immediately, steps were taken to pasteurize the supply to kill the infecting organisms before they were able to reach more potential victims. A search for the carrier among the employees of the firm, including the 12 roundsmen, was unsuccessful. Investigations spread to the thirty-seven farms that produced the milk to be mixed and distributed by the firm under suspicion. At one farm the housewife was ill with enteric fever; she died and her son developed the disease. This farm contributed 91 litres (20 gallons) of milk each day to the mixed supply of the retailer. Yet there was another puzzling feature in that a number of people had been infected before the farmer's wife became ill.

Further inquiries revealed the fact that, some years ago, a fatal case of typhoid fever had occurred in a house adjoining the farm. The water supply was common to both houses, eight others in the vicinity and also to the dairies. It came from a deep well situated about 91 metres (100 yards) from a small stream. This stream was liable to pollution from storm water and the sewage effluent from a large house. Typhoid bacilli were found in the effluent and their origin traced to a carrier in the house.

It was next demonstrated, by chemical means, that there was a connection between the stream water and the well. Furthermore, the farmer's cows and those of another producer, who also contributed to the same dealer's milk supply, used pasture alongside the stream. They drank from the stream, and perhaps while standing in it their udders were washed by the contaminated water. Spread of infection was considered to be water borne to the cows followed by contamination of the raw mixed milk supply consumed by the population. The milk was thought to have been contaminated with typhoid bacilli for 31 days before pasteurization was adopted.

Ice-cream

Before the ice-cream heat treatment Regulations were introduced in 1947, ice-cream was a common vehicle for outbreaks of food poisoning and food-borne disease. The ice-cream mix was usually contaminated during preparation and it was often stored for hours or even overnight; there was opportunity for bacterial growth, which was necessary for staphylococci to produce enterotoxin, but not so necessary for the typhoid bacillus which can cause infection in smaller numbers.

The Aberystwyth outbreak

The Aberystwyth outbreak illustrates the widespread and serious nature of an infectious disease initiated by a symptomless urinary excreter, unaware of his condition, handling a commodity such as ice-cream; he had been ill with typhoid fever in 1938 and was declared 'free of typhoid' when he recovered.

There were approximately 210 cases, with 4 deaths. Because of warm weather and holiday makers there was an increased demand for ice-cream and the merchant deviated from his usual practice of heating the ice-cream mix immediately before cooling and freezing, using instead a cold mix method which required no heat treatment of the rehydrated powdered mix. There was no indication of the time between mixing and freezing in the report of the outbreak, but the atmospheric temperature was high.

Another ice-cream outbreak with paratyphoid bacilli as the causal agent occurred in Devon.

Paratyphoid fever at a holiday resort

At a North Devon holiday resort, cases of paratyphoid fever occurred occasionally from year to year amongst holiday makers who visited the long sandy beach. As most of them had bathed at one particular end of the beach it was assumed that paratyphoid bacilli discharged into the sea from the main sewer at a point not far from the bathers were responsible. The bacteriologist who had been in charge of the investigation was not happy with this explanation and decided to find out the true source of the organisms. He suspended cotton-wool swabs attached to suitable lengths of string at various points in the main sewer, its tributaries, and finally in the sewage waste from individual houses. When he examined these swabs in the laboratory, he found that one house only was responsible for the discharge of the infecting organisms, and that a local ice-cream manufacturer and his wife lived in the house. Specimens of stool were examined from each of them and it was revealed that, although the ice-cream manufacturer himself was clear, his wife was a carrier. Their ice-cream barrow was often seen on the bathing beach, and it is likely, therefore, that small doses of paratyphoid bacilli in ice-cream from the hands of the vendor or his wife were responsible for the outbreak of paratyphoid fever, rather than the presence of paratyphoid bacilli in the sewage which discharged into the sea.

Food

Canned meat and typhoid fever

An outbreak of typhoid fever in 1954 was traced to the consumption of canned ox-tongue, and for the first time it was postulated that the typhoid bacilli were already present within the can when it was opened.

There seemed no other explanation because those persons who had handled the tongue after removal from the can were not excreters. The Argentine establishment responsible for packing the tongue used untreated water from the river de la Plata to cool the cans after processing and typhoid bacilli of the same phage type were isolated from the river.

After this event the water was chlorinated in this establishment until 1963 when the plant broke down and again untreated water was used until in 1964 there was more trouble. Evidence pointed to a can from the same place setting up a trail of contamination amongst cold cooked meats sold in a small supermarket in Scotland.

Under strict hygienic conditions the outbreak which ensued might have been confined to those who ate the meat from the one can assumed to be contaminated. Instead the organisms spread from meat to meat and about 400 case records indicated that for 3 weeks cold meats were bought by persons who subsequently became ill with typhoid fever. This spread and lingering of the organisms in the environment of the cold meat counter was encouraged by a number of factors. The can opener, slicing machine, pedestals for window shows, price tickets and trays for storage overnight in the refrigerator were common to all canned meats opened and sliced during the day. The slicing machine was washed each day but the use of plastic buckets for cloths, and of wooden scrubbing brushes in water without disinfectant may well have spread the organism without destroying it. With closure of the cold meat counter and finally of the shop itself the cases ceased to occur.

In 1963 three outbreaks of typhoid fever were all connected with canned meat from another establishment, where the cooling water was not chlorinated. One outbreak occurred after eating canned corned beef sold from a small butcher's shop with a chill cabinet. The number of cases almost coincided with the number of portions of corned beef from one pack. The sale of corned beef was stopped. The other two outbreaks occurred from canned corned beef sold by supermarkets, both with a high standard of hygiene and plentiful use of refrigerators.

As a result of these five outbreaks a careful search was made through the records of earlier outbreaks of typhoid fever. Many were said to have occurred due to cold meats bought at provision stores or butchers' shops; in every instance it had been assumed that the meat was contaminated after removal from the can. Since no symptomless excreters were found, it is probable that trace leakage of cooling water through seams had occurred during the cooling of the cans after heat processing.

Typhoid bacilli neither produce gas nor spoil the meat even though they grow abundantly in corned beef under both aerobic and anaerobic conditions. As their presence is not necessarily manifested in the blowing of contaminated cans, chlorination of water for the cooling process at canning factories should be strictly enforced.

The pease pudding outbreak of dysentery

It was customary in a certain little provisions store to prepare pease pudding one day each week. On a certain occasion several people in the vicinity of the shop were taken ill with dysentery, and inquiry revealed that they had all eaten pease pudding prepared at the little shop. Suspicions were confirmed when remains of the pudding collected from the shop were shown to contain dysentery bacilli. It was some time before the investigators were able to find out how the organisms reached the pudding. Gradually the story was pieced together. On the day that the pudding was made two visitors came to the shop, a nursemaid and her charge— a little girl 3 to 4 years of age. The nurse was a friend of a young girl who worked in the kitchen and, as was her habit, she went into the kitchen to talk to her, taking the child with her. While the two girls chatted together the child grew bored and wandered round the kitchen. Suddenly she noticed the pease pudding on the table and, deciding that it looked good to eat, she seized a handful and crammed it into her mouth. The hole in the pudding and the evidence on the child's face was vividly remembered by both the nurse and her friend. The child had recently recovered from an attack of diarrhoea which had been caused by the same dysentery bacillus as that responsible for the outbreak. The organisms were still present in her stools and must, on that occasion, have been present on her hands also, and by this means the bacilli were transferred to the pudding.

The thorough investigation of an outbreak of food poisoning may involve, therefore, not only a knowledge of the habits and illnesses of those actually employed as food handlers, but of their visitors also.

PART 2

Food Hygiene in the Prevention of Food Poisoning

9
Introduction

The previous chapters have described the bacterial causes of food poisoning, characteristics of the agents responsible, the sources or reservoirs of these germs and the conditions which encourage them to grow and reach numbers that are dangerous to the health of those who eat them.

Food hygiene may be defined as the sanitary science which aims to produce food which is safe for the consumer and of good keeping quality. It covers a wide field and includes the rearing, feeding, marketing and slaughter of animals as well as the sanitation procedures designed to prevent bacteria of human origin reaching foodstuffs. The veterinary and manufacturing aspects are beyond the scope of this book and although mentioned they are not considered in detail. With an acceptance of the fact that raw materials may contain food poisoning organisms, what can the food handler do to prevent food poisoning?

Some of the means by which foodstuffs can be protected from gross contamination will be obvious, but others may not be quite so clear. The immediate application of methods to raise standards of hygiene are sometimes thought to be impracticable, yet they should be discussed in the light of plans for future establishments designed for the preparation and service of food and for the training of food handlers.

There are two salient features which are important.

1. *The separation of raw and cooked foods* in the general work flow of the large kitchen; this includes the necessity for different areas, workers, equipment and utensils for raw ingredients and for the cooked products. Food handlers in small kitchens can only take note of the necessity for care in cleansing hands, equipment and utensils in between work with raw and cooked foods. This injunction is necessary for shops also.

2. *The care of foods after cooking* by almost any method; it is essential to cool quickly and refrigerate all foods which are not to be eaten hot and freshly cooked.

If these two measures alone were understood and taken into earnest consideration there would be little food poisoning today. Other points which are better known may be listed as follows:

(a) Care of the hands by washing is usually applied to measures to be taken after using the WC but hands should be washed carefully between work jobs and after touching raw foods.

(b) Care not to touch cooked foods with the bare hands because the washing of hands cannot be an assurance against the removal of staphylococci.

(c) The removal from work with susceptible foods of any worker with septic lesions anywhere on the body. Clean (non-suppurative abrasions) should be covered with waterproof dressings or Newskin.

(d) The elimination of flies, rats, mice and other pests from food establishments.

(e) Careful instructions for cleaning the environment, equipment, food and drink containers and utensils. Recommendations for good detergents, for cleaning and for boiling and very hot water for 'sterilization'; chemical bactericidal agents may be necessary in some instances. The substitution of disposable paper for cloths, which otherwise should be boiled daily along with mop heads used for cleaning.

The words 'food hygiene' are usually associated with personal cleanliness which is often linked with the care of the hands. Normal washing procedures will not free the hands of all bacteria; staphylococci and similar organisms will remain in pores and crevices in the skin. The mass of bacteria and food-poisoning germs picked up from raw meat and poultry can largely be washed from the hands although normal skin flora will remain. Thus care is needed not to handle cooked foods and particularly meats, poultry, custards and creams without utensils, or without disposable gloves. Yet, however carefully the food handler washes bacteria from the hands, raw products will spread them in the environment so that two more important preventive measures are: (f) cleanliness of all the surfaces and equipment used for cooked foods, and (g) rapid cooling and cold storage of foods not intended to be eaten immediately on arrival or after cooking. Thus, not only should cooked foodstuffs be protected against direct contamination by human, animal or insect vectors of bacteria but also against indirect contamination from raw foods and articles and surfaces used for preparation. The conditions of storage should ensure that foods can be kept at temperatures which will inhibit the growth and multiplication of bacteria. Cool and cold stores should be readily accessible to preparation areas. Most people will not be infected clinically by small numbers of food poisoning bacteria but when millions develop in food, resistance to infection may be overcome and sufficient toxin formed in food or intestine to cause symptoms.

All those who work with food should be made aware of the ever present yet unseen danger of contamination, and taught how to store foods which encourage bacterial multiplication so that growth is suppressed. They require knowledge of the cooking times and temperatures known to kill bacterial cells, and an awareness of the survival of some spores and toxins in spite of cooking procedures that give palatable food.

The precautions needed for the care of food after cooking with regard to methods of cooling and storage when the food is required cold and for reheating, where this is essential, must be taught in detail with strong emphasis on the ease with which bacteria from hands, surfaces, equipment and utensils can reach food after cooking. It cannot be stated too often that the design of factories, shops and kitchens should be such that raw and cooked food materials are well separated and all surfaces, implements and vessels used for foods are designed and constructed so that cleaning is easy.

The following chapters describe in more detail the measures which will lessen the risk of food poisoning; these factors have been recognized while studying the spread of infection both in the field of outbreaks and in the laboratory.

There are other factors, sometimes magnified in the public mind, which may be relatively unimportant in themselves and which may serve merely as an indication that the conditions in a particular establishment are not all that may be desired. The presence of lipstick on a cup is not necessarily a sign that dangerous germs must be present also, but that the washing-up has not been carried out with due care and attention. Varnish on the nails of a waitress or kitchen employee is not in itself a harbour for bacteria, but perhaps an indication that the hands will not be washed or the nails scrubbed as often as required, for fear of damaging the cosmetic effect. The flakes of whitewash which may fall from the ceiling into food during its preparation may not constitute an immediate danger, but indicate that the general care of the kitchen is poor. The much-handled unwrapped loaf will not give rise to food poisoning or even food-borne infection except in quite unusual circumstances, yet it indicates a lack of care and respect for the food which others have to eat.

There are many such examples which arouse feelings of apprehension in the minds of people and which perhaps divert attention from more serious lapses in personal habits such as fingering the nose and mouth with hands used for the preparation of foods, failure to wash the hands between and after jobs, which include work with raw foodstuffs, as well as the after-care of cooked foods cut up for the table or to be cooled and stored.

The remaining chapters on prevention are concerned with the food handler, the food itself, the environment and equipment of food premises, and the parts which can be played by education and legislation.

10
Personal Hygiene of the Food Handler

There is a chain of events which links the human or animal carrier or temporary excreter of food-poisoning bacteria to the food and subsequently encourages the organisms to multiply in the food before it reaches the victim. Every food producer and food handler has a part to play in the application of hygienic practices so that the links in this chain of infection may be broken.

Care of the hands

The passage of bacteria from one food to another on the hands of the food handler is an important means of spread with the hands providing a way of transport. There are personal skin bacteria which cling to the skin surface and persist in hair follicles, pores, crevices and lesions caused by breaks in the skin. It is extremely difficult and perhaps impossible to remove these organisms by normal hand washing methods. When *Staphylococcus aureus* joins the population of the skin flora, there is danger from the contamination of food by those who finger foods in the course of preparation (see Fig. 8).

Merely eating a few hundreds, or even thousands, of staphylococcal cells newly planted on cooked food will be harmless. The number of organisms must increase to many millions per gram of food during unchilled storage for sufficient toxin to be formed in the food to give symptoms of sickness.

Organisms habitually found in the bowel and which may pass through porous toilet paper, or be picked up from raw meat and poultry, can be washed more readily from the hands than those of the inherent skin flora. Experiments with salmonellae implanted on fingers and allowed to dry have indicated that there is a steady reduction in numbers but that there are usually a few survivors after 3 hours; when the original number was small they disappeared more rapidly. In these experiments a good hand wash removed these organisms.

The hands should be washed with plenty of soap and warm water and preferably rinsed in running water. Nails should be kept short, unvarnished and scrupulously clean. Nail brushes should be made of plastic with Nylon bristles which may be disinfected periodically, preferably by heat or in a hypochlorite solution; a nail file should be available. Intestinal as well as skin and nose food-poisoning bacteria have been isolated from swabs rubbed under the nails.

Soap dispensed from a fixed container in a liquid or finely flaked or powdered form has advantages over soap tablets. When passed from hand to hand soap may accumulate a scum and curd thereby trapping bacteria which can remain on the surface. Tablets should be kept in a dry dish or suspended from a bracket by means of a small magnet. While liquid soap may have advantages it can be a breeding ground for bacteria unless it contains a disinfectant. Soaps containing bactericidal substances are available in liquid or tablet form. The exclusive and prolonged use of antiseptic soaps may reduce the bacterial flora of the hands, and the repeated use of bactericidal liquid soap has been shown to reduce the distribution of hand contaminants.

Investigations on the bacterial flora of hands before and after washing with soap and water, alone or supplemented by antiseptic treatment, on a short-term basis showed that soap and water were effective in reducing or removing coliform organisms acquired from foods. The resident population of staphylococci, although reduced, may still be found on the hands after washing; they lodge in the hair follicles and cracks of the skin and may come to the surface after scrubbing in hot water. It is difficult to alter the resident flora of the hands, thus washed hands do not necessarily mean safe hands. Foods which readily support the growth of staphylococci for example, cooked meats, cured and uncured, creams, and cooked seafoods, should not be touched with the fingers.

Food handlers touch equipment and utensils as well as foodstuffs, and pass on micro-organisms as well as acquiring them; therefore, care should be taken with the handling of equipment used in the preparation of food. Many food manufacturing establishments now dispense creams and lotions containing bactericidal substances for use after hand washing, in an effort to reduce the numbers of bacteria passing from hand to food when procedures cannot be performed by machine. Plain barrier creams decrease the sensitivity of hands to the effect of some food substances which have been known to produce dermatitis in certain people; they also keep the hands soft and supple so that roughness and cracks which may

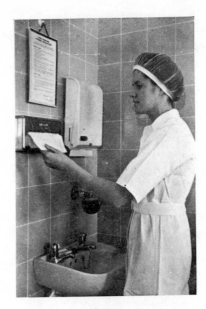

Fig. 19.   Paper towel and tissues;
            practical head-dress

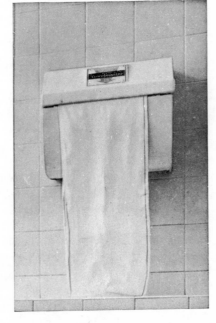

Fig. 20.   Continuous roller towel

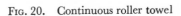

harbour bacteria are prevented. Barrier creams may contain a disinfectant in order to prevent growth of bacteria in the cream.

Tests have indicated that the use of rubber gloves is not necessarily an improvement bacteriologically over the use of bare hands unless the gloves retain a smooth unbroken surface and are washed frequently. They should be washed inside as well as outside

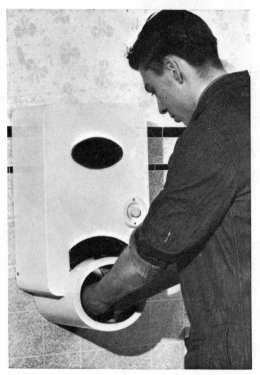

FIG. 21.   Hot-air dryer

to prevent soiling the hands by wearing gloves after continual use. The use of gloves is recommended, however, for procedures involving frozen foods and also when there is prolonged immersion of the hands in hot water containing detergents; in such instances protection of the skin is advisable. Thin disposable gloves are available for light work with foods, such as the assembly of salads; they should not be worn for too long. Care should be taken to avoid irritating substances, unnecessary contact with dirt, chapping, or contact with very hot water.

Disposable paper towels are probably the most satisfactory means for drying the hands (Fig. 19). Alternatively, cloth towels issued individually for each person's use and regularly laundered are acceptable. The continuous roller towel system (Fig. 20) which provides a portion of clean towel for each person is far better than the communal roller towel. The use of communal towels should be discontinued; they have been known to transfer infection from one person to another. It is almost impossible, even in the smallest establishment, to ensure that the hands are dried on a previously

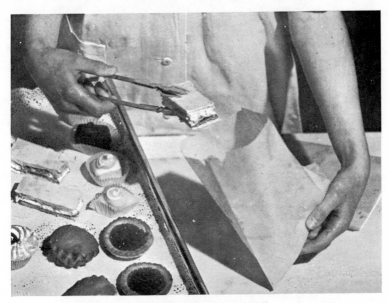

FIG. 22.   Pastry tongs

unsoiled portion of a roller towel, except by making extravagant demands on the laundering services. Electric hot-air dryers are pleasant to use, but they require more time (Fig. 21).

As already stressed, the skin of the hands must be kept not only clean but soft and healthy. A simple and inexpensive hand lotion may be made from gum tragacanth and glycerin in the proportion of one part of tragacanth to two parts of glycerin in water with the addition of a few drops each of the oils of lemon and lavender; there are also commercially produced hand creams which are both effective and economical.

Cuts, burns and other raw surfaces however small and healthy looking can harbour staphylococci; there is a compulsory measure imposed by the Food Hygiene (General) Regulations, 1970, that in the kitchen all lesions must be covered. Waterproof dressings are essential to prevent the passage of bacteria outwards in the serous fluid or inwards from fluids in the environment. When a lesion is obviously infected as shown by inflammation

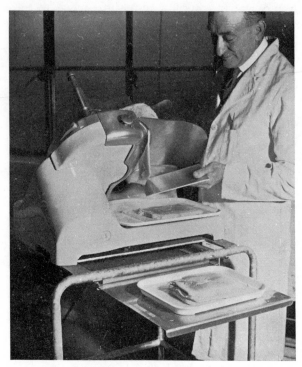

Fig. 23.   Hygienic method of slicing meat

and pus formation, whether it be on the hand or on any other part of the body, the person concerned should not handle foods. Even when the lesion has healed it should be remembered that the infecting staphylococci may still linger in the skin of the hands and that they may be difficult to eliminate. Skin disease from some other cause may be colonized by staphylococci so that care should be taken with skin conditions such as dermatitis from foods. The resident population of staphylococci, although reduced, may still be found on the hands after washing; they lodge in the hair follicles and cracks of the skin and may come to the surface after scrubbing in hot water. It is difficult to alter the resident flora of the hands.

It is important, therefore, to remember that foods should not be touched with the bare hands more than is absolutely necessary. There is far too much handling of susceptible foodstuffs not only in kitchens but also in the retail shop and factory. It should be possible to have implements to carry out the work of the fingers, particularly with meat and confectionery that are not to be cooked subsequently. It may be slower to use tongs rather than fingers to serve cream cakes and sandwiches and to manoeuvre sliced meat from a machine but the extra time may be a factor in the prevention of food poisoning (Figs. 22 and 23).

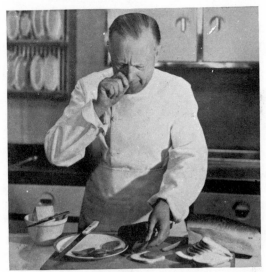

Fig. 24.   Habits to avoid—fingering the nose while preparing sandwiches

Habits

There are certain bad habits which should be avoided by the food handler. The unguarded cough or sneeze can disperse from the nose, mouth or throat numbers of bacteria suspended in droplets of moisture. These droplets serve to pass infection directly from one person to another; they may also contaminate foodstuffs.

The habit of licking the fingers to pick up paper or to turn over the pages of a book is a bad one at any time but particularly so when the paper, contaminated with saliva, is used for wrapping food.

Nose picking or fingering the nose may leave staphylococci or other harmful organisms on the fingers. Clean handkerchiefs are almost free from bacteria, but dirty ones may harbour many millions; paper handkerchiefs provide a more hygienic substitute for cloth. The disposal of paper handkerchiefs should not create a problem; they may be flushed individually down the water closet or burned in a sanitary incinerator, or collected in a pedal-operated bin kept for the purpose and subsequently incinerated.

The hair should be clean and kept tidy by means of a cap, net or head-scarf (Fig. 19); hair and dandruff can spread staphylococci from lesions on the scalp. The use of tobacco in any form is prohibited under the Food Hygiene Regulations so that smoking while on duty must be avoided. Smoke and ash from a cigarette are harmless but many smokers contaminate their fingers with saliva while taking the cigarette from their lips or when removing loose pieces of tobacco from the mouth. Other habits, such as chewing gum and taking snuff, which may result in the contamination of the fingers and environment should also be discouraged.

It is the practice in many self-service restaurants to clean table-tops with a moist cloth, when the crockery has been cleared away. The water used for rinsing the cloths should contain a suitable quantity of hypochlorite, or a quaternary ammonium compound or other bactericidal substance, and the cloths themselves should be boiled and dried overnight or steeped in hypochlorite. For preference, paper should be used. Forks, spoons, cups and glasses should be handled correctly by keeping the fingers from those parts which are touched by food and the mouth. Cutlery kept in a communal box should be supplied wrapped in a paper napkin.

Intestinal execreters

Intestinal bacteria are more likely to spread from the fluid stools excreted by those with diarrhoea than from the well-formed stools of the normal person. Aerosol sprays when the WC is flushed and general toilet cleanliness are more difficult with fluid excreta. Those with diarrhoea should not work in the kitchen, whatever job they are doing. Clearance from intestinal pathogens is required for food handlers under the Food Hygiene Regulations. The treatment of healthy excreters with antibiotics is not recommended because it may prolong the period of excretion.

The spread of intestinal pathogens, such as salmonellae in hospital wards may be particularly troublesome. Nurses taking bedpans from bed to bed, the disposal of excreta in sluice rooms not far away from the ward followed by the dispensation of meals in the same area by nurses and patients raises peculiar difficulties in control.

Clothes, illnesses and education

Protective clothing should be light coloured and changed frequently. Modern drip-dry fabrics ease the work of daily laundering. The provision of shower-baths in changing rooms will encourage a high standard of personal cleanliness. All large establishments should be provided with adequate changing rooms, rest rooms and provision for storing clothes and other personal belongings. Illnesses, however mild, should be reported at once to the medical department and those which are likely to give rise to the spread of bacteria known to cause food poisoning or sepsis are required to be notified to the medical officer of health. Most large shops, stores and factories possess a well equipped medical department including a surgery and waiting room. Small shops and kitchens should possess a first-aid box, and keep at least one member of the staff up to date in first-aid treatment.

Education on good standards of health and hygiene for all those working with food should be provided by the medical officer, public health inspector, welfare nurse or other responsible person, and regular talks should be encouraged.

11

Storage and Preparation and Retail Shops

Ways in which the food handler can help to prevent food poisoning have been discussed in the previous chapter. Yet without facilities to aid rapid cooling and to store foods under cold conditions, bacteria will multiply to dangerous levels and there may be accumulation of toxic substances.

STORAGE

Cold storage

Cold affects micro-organisms in different ways depending on its intensity. As the temperature falls, bacterial activity declines; therefore foods which support bacterial growth should be stored at low temperatures to prolong their life and maintain safety. When foods are 'chilled' or stored at temperatures near but above freezing point some bacteria will grow slowly, but in the frozen or solid state many micro-organisms will be killed directly in the process of freezing; the remainder will not multiply and the numbers tend gradually to diminish. Hence freezing preserves foods for a long time, while chilling merely delays decomposition for a week or so.

Chilled storage

In the refrigeration trade the term 'chilling' is used to cover any reduction in the normal temperature of the article concerned. For example, the ripening of tropical fruits is delayed during transit by storage at a temperature not far below that of the atmosphere, whereas the decomposition of imported meat is delayed by storage at -3 to $1\,°C$ ($26\cdot6$ to $33\cdot8\,°F$) on the ship.

Some foods cannot be chilled at too low a temperature because there may be harmful changes; for instance, the inside flesh of apples turns brown if chilled below $3\cdot5\,°C$ ($38\cdot3\,°F$) and the resistance of some fruits to moulds may be destroyed by chilling, so that the rate of spoilage by moulds is increased.

136

With regard to pathogenic organisms some strains of salmonellae will grow at 10 °C (50 °F) but not at 5 °C (41 °F). Staphylococci will not grow below about 10 °C (50 °F); at 20 °C (68 °F) there is growth and toxin production. The sporing anaerobic organism, *Clostridium welchii*, will not grow at temperatures much below 15 to 20 °C (59 to 68 °F), and no growth was observed in 6 days at 6·5 °C (43·7 °F). Most species of *Cl. botulinum* will grow very slowly at 10 °C (50 °F) and in some instances toxins may be formed at this temperature; in general, there is no growth or toxin formation at 5 °C (41 °F) although one species, type E, not only grows at 3·5 °C (38·3 °F) but produces toxin also.

Many other bacteria are able to increase slowly at chill temperatures, and under prolonged domestic refrigeration at 4 to 5 °C (39·2 to 41·0 °F) they will gradually spoil foods. Milk, for example, will develop off-flavours and off-odours from the growth of bacteria better adapted to the cold than those which grow and sour the milk at normal temperatures.

Foods of good bacteriological quality may be kept in a satisfactory condition at 4 °C for 3 to 4 days.

Deep freeze storage

The freezing of foodstuffs at approximately − 18 °C (0 °F) kills many organisms, and the rate of death of the remainder will depend partly on the temperature of storage. Of the food-poisoning organisms, those of the salmonella group are said to disappear most rapidly on freezing. It has been reported that salmonella organisms disappear in 1 month and staphylococci in 5 months from strawberries kept at − 18 °C (0 °F). Yet salmonellae have been isolated after years of frozen storage in whole egg products and meat. The spores of *Cl. welchii* and *Cl. botulinum* are not affected by freezing and the poisonous toxin of *Cl. botulinum* has considerable resistance to alternate freezing and thawing at a temperature as low as − 50 °C (− 58 °F). Staphylococcal enterotoxin has been shown to withstand a temperature of − 4 °C (24·8 °F) for 2 months.

Moulds and yeasts endure freezing conditions better than bacteria, thus refrigerators should be kept thoroughly cleaned and free from fungal and yeast growth.

When highly contaminated foodstuffs are kept frozen it is believed that changes may occur in the food owing to the slow activity of surviving organisms over a long period of time. Thus there may be slow spoilage during storage in the frozen state, although far less, of course, than that which would occur in the unfrozen food. Chemical changes in enzyme structures may also take place. Freezing will not restore the freshness of a food already highly contaminated or spoiled by bacterial action. When a frozen food is thawed those bacteria which have survived will recommence growth and decomposition, so that the keeping time of the food is limited and it must not be left at room temperature too long before eating, nor should it be refrozen. Manufacturers take great care in the preparation of frozen foods and most of them print instructions on the packet for their correct use. A temporary period of thawing due to power cuts or failure of the cabinet mechanism or even during shopping does not necessarily mean that the partially thawed food should be discarded. Discretion must be used depending on the length of time, rise in temperature and general condition of the food. When the central core is still frozen the outside will still be cold enough to stop most bacteria from growing. Frozen food should be eaten as the manufacturer intends, freshly thawed from the original frozen state. Subsequent thawing and freezing will lead to quality deterioration as well as bacterial hazard.

Cold storage accommodation

There should be ample cold storage space conveniently available in every kitchen. Where the size of the canteen justifies the extra expense there should be a walk-in cold room with metal shelves and, in addition, one or more household refrigerators, so that foods with strong odours, such as fish, may be kept separate from other foods. Between the cold room and the kitchen there should be a well defined air space to prevent the hot air from the kitchen reaching the cold room. The temperatures of all domestic refrigerators and cold rooms should be checked regularly by thermometers placed in positions where they can be read easily. Cold rooms and domestic refrigerators are usually maintained at temperatures from 1 to 4 °C (33·8 to 39·2 °F).

The life of food in the refrigerator is limited and the longer it remains there the shorter its life on removal. The results of experiments on the storage life at 0 °C of meat with different initial numbers of bacteria indicated that meat of good bacteriological quality before refrigeration would keep for many days whereas poor quality meat had a short storage life. When the initial count of bacteria was low the appearance of slime on refrigerated meat was delayed for 18 days; when counts were high before refrigeration, slime appeared in 8 days. Conditions for the temporary storage of various foodstuffs are recommended by the Ministry of Agriculture, Fisheries and Food (p.152); similar recommendations are given in the United States of America (Fig. 57, p. 256).

Refrigerators should be defrosted regularly, automatically or according to the manufacturer's instructions. They should not be over-crowded, so that air circulation may be good; it is advisable to check the contents at the time of defrosting and aged foods should be thrown away. Space in the refrigerator ought to be available for cooked and uncooked foods which are perishable because they are susceptible to bacterial attack, such as meat, poultry, egg and dairy products and fish. Tinfoil, greaseproof paper or Polythene wrapped around foods will prevent loss of moisture and the spread of flavours to other foods. Many foodstuffs commonly stored in a refrigerator do not encourage bacterial growth and they can with safety be kept for a few days in a cool room on a slate or stone slab; for example, fats, such as lard, margarine and butter, hard cheese, unopened canned goods, cured bacon and shell eggs. Milk can be stored in the cool room during the winter, but in the summer it should be refrigerated whether in bottles or churns. Receptacles containing milk should be covered and the outside cleaned before they are placed in the refrigerator, cold room or larder.

At the time of defrosting, walls and shelves should be washed with soap or detergent and warm water and carefully dried before the food is replaced. If refrigerators are switched off at holiday times they must be emptied and carefully dried to prevent mould growth.

Domestic refrigerators are intended to keep food cold, and not to cool hot food which may damage the cooling coils and cause moisture to condense on adjacent cold foods; this may encourage the growth of slime bacteria and moulds. Cooked foods should, therefore, be cooled rapidly and placed in the refrigerator within $1\frac{1}{2}$ hours of cooking. An exception might be made for placing hot food in a walk-in type of cold room.

The penetration of heat into large joints and the loss of heat after cooking are slow, so that cuts of meat should be limited in size to 2·7 kg (6 lb) or less unless special precautions are taken for cooling in a chilled atmosphere with a good circulation of air.

Cooling rates

The rapid cooling of bulks of cooked food intended to be eaten hours or even days later presents difficulties. The results of experiments to estimate the cooling rate of large cuts of meat showed that immediate storage in a well ventilated cold room was the most effective method; 2·3 kg (5 lb) cuts of meat lost approximately 60° of heat, cooling from 70 to 10°C (158 to 50°F) in 1½ to 2 hours. In homes and small catering establishments when cool rooms may not be available hot meat should be left in a cool and draughty place for not longer than 1½ hours before refrigeration. Even so storage of large cuts of meat cooked by boiling or by other methods not requiring temperatures above 100°C should be discouraged.

Some food factories cool by wind-tunnels measuring about 1·5 by 0·9 by 24·4 metres long (5 by 3 by 80 feet) provided with iron rails, and while the food on metal trays passes through it is subjected to the wind from a fan 1·5 to 2 metres (60 to 80 inches) in diameter; cupboards with descending cold air-streams are also used. For large establishments compelled to cool masses of food required for frozen or chilled meals a mechanism should be provided to keep a cooling room at 10°C (50°F). Some new kitchens for school canteens include this facility; it is hoped that in time accommodation for efficient cooling will be provided in all kitchens cooking for large numbers of people. For small establishments a simple circulating fan installed in a well ventilated cooling room or larder situated on the north side of the building will provide a satisfactory system. A cabinet with shelves and containing a fan and air filter has been designed for quick cooling. Shallow rather than deep containers provide a larger cooling area for stews, gravies and other liquid foods prepared in bulk. Household refrigerators could be adapted to provide space for shallow trays stacked one above the other for the cold storage of liquids.

Improvised cooling

Most houses and flats possess a cool cupboard or larder fitted with slate or stone slabs and with a ventilator protected against flies. Where the air flow is limited a small fan would be helpful. Foods should be covered, but all materials must allow an exchange of air otherwise there will be an increase in humidity, which will encourage mould and bacterial growth. Where space for cool storage is not available a box, louvered to allow a free flow of air but protected from rain, should be hung on a north wall or, at least, out of the sun.

There are various improvised methods for keeping food cool in the home. Porous earthenware vessels cooled with water help to keep foods such as milk and butter cold by evaporation. Muslin covering a bottle of milk or other container may be kept damp by dipping the four corners in cold water held in an outer receptacle; the container should be placed in a draught and out of the sun. A small louvered cupboard standing in water contained in a large basin or bath may be used for more bulky foods. Milk delivered after a family leaves for work should be placed in an insulated box, such as a polystyrene container, kept by the door in the shade.

Frozen packs of food allowed to thaw should be cooked and eaten within a short time; a vacuum flask will keep frozen foods solid for an extra day and delay the growth of bacteria for 3 to 4 days. The polystyrene container designed particularly to keep ice-cream solid is effective over a shorter period of time than the vacuum flask but it will delay the growth of bacteria for at least 24 hours.

Frozen meals for elderly incapacitated folk living alone may be stored in either of these containers for 2 to 3 days after delivery.

In the UK the summer temperatures vary between 18 and 20 °C (64 and 69 °F) with occasional heatwaves with temperatures up to 32 °C (90 °F). Winter temperatures are usually 1 to 5 °C (35 to 41 °F) with occasional cold spells, and warm days when temperatures of 10 °C (50 °F) may be recorded.

Kitchen and shop temperatures will be considerably higher.

The incidence of food poisoning is highest in the summer but cases and outbreaks occur all through the year. Adequate cold storage in all homes and shops would help to reduce the incidence of food poisoning; there is really no method which can effectively replace refrigeration.

The education of food handlers in matters of food hygiene should include instruction in the correct use of refrigerators and cold rooms. In particular they must be taught that the cleanliness and safety of a refrigerated foodstuff are dependent on the extent of bacterial contamination before refrigeration as well as on the temperature of refrigeration; also that extreme cold merely delays the growth and multiplication of bacteria, which immediately renew their activity when the food is transferred to a warm room.

Other storage

In addition to refrigerated and cool storage there should be dry, light and airy cupboards or rooms for canned and other packaged goods stacked on shelves and marked for rotation. Powdered and granular foods such as flour, sugar, dried milk, tea, oatmeal, sago, rice, egg powder and coconut should be stored in metal bins or metal or glass jars with close-fitting lids. Even these containers should be raised at least 450 mm (18 inches) above the floor to allow space for cleaning. Goods packed in cardboard or wooden crates or cases should be well clear of the floor and preferably on higher shelves. The rooms should be designed to discourage vermin, flies and dust and they should be easy to clean.

Vegetables should be stored and prepared in a separate room or section of the kitchen so that dust and earth from potatoes, carrots, turnips and other root vegetables may be diverted from areas of food preparation.

Cleaning materials also require separate cupboards or small rooms. Personal clothing and other belongings should not be left in the kitchen but in proper accommodation provided nearby.

Equipment for cooking, receptacles, utensils, crockery and cutlery, should be stacked and protected from dust.

PREPARATION AND COOKING

Fresh food cooked and eaten immediately while hot should never be responsible for food poisoning due to micro-organisms. Nevertheless, heat-resistant bacterial spores frequently survive cooking and give rise to large numbers of bacterial cells when cooling is slow and the storage time of cooked foods in the kitchen is too long.

Short, high-temperature cooking is best for the safety of the food-stuff and thereafter there must be an understanding of times and temperatures of storage in relation to bacterial growth.

Steam under pressure, thorough roasting of small solid chunks of meat, grilling and frying are considered to be the safest methods of cooking. Infra-red rays and high-frequency waves have good penetration but may be patchy in action. The results of comparative experiments with small chickens inoculated with sporing and non-sporing organisms showed that some spores survived inside and on the outer surfaces of the carcasses after cooking in a microwave oven and also after conventional roasting. Both methods of cooking destroyed vegetative cells. The rapid reheating of chilled or thawed frozen meals in a microwave oven may have advantages in some circumstances and for certain foods, but the bacteriological condition of the cooked food before reheating is important. All the benefit of heat destruction of micro-organisms in raw food by cooking may be undone if manipulation and handling after heating allows recontamination of the cooked food.

Meat and poultry dishes

Heat penetrates slowly into joints, poultry carcasses and made-up dishes such as pies, and adequate cooking times and temperatures should be allowed for the centre to reach boiling point. For instance, a 2·9 kg (6½ lb) meat pie requires a temperature of 177 to 204 °C (350 to 400 °F) for 2½ to 3 hours for the centre to reach boiling point at 100 °C (212 °F). An outbreak of food poisoning has already been described in which an organism of the salmonella group was isolated from several pies of two sizes; 453 and 113 g (1 lb and 4 oz). The minced meat, probably already contaminated with salmonellae, was hand-filled raw into the pastry cases and it was thought that the cooking, at 232 to 246 °C (450 to 475 °F) for 25 to 30 minutes, was either inadequate to destroy the contaminants or that there were temperature fluctuations. It was pointed out that pies made with raw meat should be cooked to the point of sterility even though the pastry may become a little over-brown in the process. It is worth while to note that for the red muscle colouring matter of meat to change to the familiar grey colour the temperature must be at least 73 °C (163·4 °F). Heat penetrates meat slowly and the English roast beef which remains red inside has not reached an internal temperature of more than 63 to 65 °C (145·4 to 149 °F). Slowly cooked rare beef used for sandwiches prepared for customers at their request has caused *Cl. welchii* food poisoning.

Precooked meat is often used for making pies and pasties so that a final cooking time sufficient only to bake the pastry is given. The temperature reached in the centre of the mass of meat, sometimes mixed with vegetables, would not necessarily destroy sporing or even non-sporing organisms which would multiply actively while the meat was still warm.

In 1969, 39 of 189 (21 per cent) outbreaks of food poisoning in hospitals, schools, institutions, restaurants and canteens were due to *Cl. welchii* and the foods most commonly mentioned were cold or reheated meat and poultry and meat pies made with precooked meat. Thus a change in cooking and storage techniques would help to eliminate this type of food poisoning.

Part-cooking of meat in hot weather or at any other time is frowned on by the bacteriologist. Some organisms will be killed but others may be encouraged to multiply. The final cooking may be too light either to kill bacteria or to destroy toxins.

It is safer to keep meat in the raw state overnight, preferably in the cold, and to cook it thoroughly on the day when it is required. If, from motives of economy or for some other reason, it is essential to cook meat the day before it is eaten, it should be cooked thoroughly, cooled rapidly and refrigerated overnight. When there is insufficient refrigerator space, it should be a strict rule that all dishes of stewed or boiled meat, whether as stews, pies or joints, must be cooked and eaten the same day, preferably with no delay between cooking and eating and certainly not more than 1 to 2 hours. The danger of eating meat and poultry cooked a day or two earlier seems to be far greater in the communal canteen dealing with large masses of meat than in the home, although in no instance should stewed or boiled meat be allowed to stand at a warm temperature for several hours. Well-roasted solid meats should be safe, but the rolled roast joint frequently gives rise to trouble because the contaminated outside is folded into the centre. The size and shape of joints of meat are important in relation to heat penetration and heat loss. Temperature recordings from thermocouples showed that during cooking the temperature at any point within the meat was dependent on the distance of that point from the outer surface of the meat. The centres of large bulky cuts of meat will, therefore, take longer to heat and cool than those of long slim portions of like weight. It was also shown experimentally that the centres of large portions of meat were slower to heat up in an hot-air oven than in a moist-air oven.

The degree of heat reached inside a grilled or fried sausage or a sausage roll will depend on the preference of the cook for a well-browned or lightly cooked article. Rissoles and fishcakes made with precooked meat or fish or potatoes, may be placed in the frying-pan or grilled for a few minutes only. Boiled rice may be quickly turned over in a little hot fat for frying. Raw foods such as fish, sliced or minced meat, and bacon are likely to be grilled or fried thoroughly on both sides in fat, which should ensure sterility.

The installation and use of pressure cookers for quick, high-temperature cooking might solve many of the difficulties associated with the preparation of foodstuffs on the day they are required to be eaten hot. Even heat-resistant spores would be killed by this method of cooking.

Canteen-prepared tongue is a frequent vehicle of *Cl. welchii* and staphylococcal food poisoning. *Cl. welchii*, from the organisms already present in the raw tongue, and staphylococci from the hands of the cooks, will multiply in the cooked product. The following method is recommended for safety. The cured tongue should be washed and allowed to soak in water for 8 hours in a cold room overnight. It should be washed well and boiled quickly in a lidded saucepan or steamer. The skin should be removed while the tongue is hot, and the small bones removed from the thick end. The tongue is then ready to be pressed in a sterilized container; at this stage it is allowed to cool, but it is cooked again in the press, cooled rapidly and refrigerated until required.

Outbreaks of poultry food poisoning frequently occur from cold or warmed poultry meat. Salmonellae and *Cl. welchii* are commonly present in the frozen or chilled birds as they arrive. The spores of *Cl. welchii* may not be destroyed by cooking and grow out later during long slow cooling and kitchen storage. Even a few salmonellae may survive in under thawed and undercooked carcasses, although they are most often picked up after cooking from traces of the raw product left on surfaces and utensils. Left unchilled, the organisms grow in the meat.

Outbreaks of salmonella food poisoning from spit-roasted chickens have been described in Chapter 6. Careful instructions are needed for thawing, cooking and, most important of all, for handling and storage of cooked poultry. Staphylococci are usually implanted by hands after cooking. Cooked carcasses may be cut and torn apart while still warm and the portions piled high on trays, so that even if refrigerated the cooling rate is far too slow. When removed from the refrigerator or cold room in good time next day the organisms continue to grow and produce toxin.

Milk foods

The hazards associated with the preparation of food a day or so ahead of requirements apply also to custards, trifles, blancmange and other milk puddings; these dishes should be freshly cooked unless they can be stored in a refrigerator.

By heating (or cooking) milk gently, as in pasteurization, all the vegetative cells of organisms which are potentially dangerous are destroyed so that the milk is made safe unless recontaminated in the home. The term 'sterilized milk' means that a temperature is reached at which all or nearly all bacteria are destroyed, and the milk will remain sterile for an indefinite period, whilst it is kept in the sealed container. Ultra heat treated milk is subjected to a high temperature by injection of steam; not all spores are destroyed but the chilled shelf-life of the milk in unopened cartons may be as long as 3 months. There have been some noteworthy episodes of food poisoning from dehydrated milk. Two outbreaks are described, one in the UK due to staphylococcal enterotoxin and the other in the USA due to *Salmonella new brunswick*.

The susceptibility of certain confectionery creams to bacterial contamination has already been emphasized, and their preparation and storage should be considered with care. All ingredients used in the vicinity should be free from pathogenic organisms and gross bacterial contamination. Equipment should be scrupulously clean and disinfected frequently. Savoy bags for dispensing cream and other toppings and also mashed potato should be made of materials which can be washed and boiled after use, such as cotton, linen or nylon. After boiling they should be dried thoroughly and stored in a special place protected from dust-borne or other contamination. Disposable paper bags may also be used for this purpose.

Although it may be considered necessary to ensure freedom from salmonellae of persons handling cream and milk, the presence of both these organisms in the cow herself may be of even greater importance. Little space has been devoted to *Brucella abortus* in cows and *Brucella melitensis* in goats but these organisms and others like the tubercle bacilli are scourges to cattle and to those who drink raw milk in countries without eradication schemes and without pasteurization. Nevertheless, the habit of boiling milk is universal.

Infant bottle feeds

Careful precautions are necessary in the preparation and storage of bottle feeds for infants. Bacteria may be introduced into prepared feeds by constituents of the feed, bottles, teats, utensils and also from hands used in the preparation. Investigations have shown that high counts may be due to bacterial growth during cooling and storage at atmospheric temperatures; unless care is taken at every stage of preparation, unsafe feeds contaminated with pathogenic bacteria and unclean feeds containing large numbers of so-called saprophytic bacteria may be given to infants.

There is a growing interest in the procedures of hospital milk kitchens and the preparation of safe infant feeds. Hospitals in the UK, in the USA and other countries are using terminal sterilization techniques. In one large hospital in India the incidence of *Esch. coli* enteritis in infants has been markedly reduced by this procedure. The cooked feed is poured into sterilized bottles; a sterilized teat is placed on each bottle and covered with a paper cap; the complete bottled feeds with teats are placed in small crates, ready for feeding each child for a day, and given heat treatment in a pressure cooker or steamer. Special equipment is available for cleaning bottles and teats (pp. 180–181).

Much care, attention and legislation have been given to the hygienic production of milk, both liquid and dried, for the general public; similar care is needed to ensure a safe clean product for the infant consumer.

Other infant feeds

Bone or meat and vegetable broths and purées are common weaning foods for infants during the second 6 months of life. The care of these foods, which may be canned or prepared in large quantities in the home, is important because they are excellent media for the growth of bacteria. The sterile contents of small bottles or cans are intended to be eaten for one meal. There are closure methods for bottles designed to prevent opening by curious mothers anxious to know the smell of the product before purchase. The preparation in the home of small quantities for individual meals may be uneconomical and large quantities may be stored for a few days only in the refrigerator.

Contaminants can be introduced from hands or from utensils, and they will grow rapidly in warm weather without refrigeration.

Infants are more sensitive than adults to food infections and more likely to succumb to the dehydration caused by diarrhoea and vomiting.

All foods and liquids intended for infants should be stored in covered containers in a refrigerator or, if canned, the portion left in the can should be refrigerated in the can and covered. Three days should be the maximum time of storage. Supplies prepared for 2 days should be separated into two portions to avoid further touching. Where there is no refrigeration the covered container should be stored in the coolest place and the food boiled immediately before the meal. When the indoor temperature is greater than 21°C (70 °F) and there is no refrigeration, bone and meat meals ought not to be used unless the contents of a freshly opened can is consumed; anything left over should be abandoned.

All containers and utensils used for the preparation of infant foods should be boiled after cleaning and allowed to drain dry (p. 181).

Egg products

Small numbers of organisms of the salmonella group may be present in unpasteurized egg products prepared in bulk, including liquid and dried whole egg, white and yolk. It is recommended that liquid egg mixes and rehydrated powders should be cooked within 2 hours of preparation unless refrigerated in small amounts. Such egg products should be used only in recipes requiring thorough heat treatment.

An outbreak of food poisoning which occurred in an army camp illustrates a number of these points. Reconstituted spray-dried whole egg was prepared early one morning; part of it was scrambled for breakfast and eaten by 70 men, only 1 of whom was affected. The portion which remained was allowed to stay in the cookhouse until tea-time when the original bacterial population, including salmonella organisms, would have increased enormously. The mixture was lightly scrambled with insufficient heat treatment to kill all the salmonellae, and of 20 men who ate it 16 were taken ill.

Infection from contaminated ducks' eggs can be avoided by boiling them hard—for at least 10 minutes—frying well on both sides or confining their use to baked products, such as cakes and puddings, which require cooking temperatures high enough to destroy the organisms. But care should be taken that all equipment used in the preparation of mixes containing ducks' eggs is thoroughly cleaned and sterilized. Outbreaks of food poisoning have been caused by the contamination of imitation cream mixed in a bowl previously used for the sponge or cake mixture containing ducks' eggs. Lightly cooked or uncooked dishes, such as scrambles, omelettes, meringues, mayonnaise, mousse or similar foods, should not be made with ducks' eggs. Other outbreaks from eggs and egg products are described in Chapter 6.

Gelatin

Powdered gelatin is another substance which requires particular care in preparation and addition to foodstuffs, because it may contain a large and varied flora of bacteria. Melted gelatin in water for use in cooked meat pies and also for other purposes such as for glazing meat loaves should be nearly boiled, and used as rapidly as possible with the temperature maintained above 60 °C (140 °F). This procedure may involve the use of a higher concentration of gelatin than formerly needed at low temperatures to produce an effective gel. Microbiological standards for the various forms of gelatin used for cooking and also for feeding animals will reduce the hazards associated with this product.

Coconut

Methods for the production of desiccated coconut are so much improved that contamination with salmonellae has been reduced to a minimum. When purchases of desiccated coconut are made from reputable firms, who know safe sources of supply, there is little danger from the use of this popular garnish. Coconut milk is sterile unless the outer husk of the nut or seed is damaged and bacteria pass through into the white flesh. Coconut milk is used as a refreshing drink in hot countries where the palm is common.

Rice

Dried polished rice has low counts of bacteria but *Bacillus cereus* is often present; this organism produces many spores which can survive cooking. The spores germinate into bacilli which multiply in cooked and moist cereal products left unrefrigerated, and a toxic substance is formed. Boiled rice intended for frying should not be stored in the kitchen, but prepared in small amounts and fried for customers as required. Outbreaks of food poisoning caused by the growth of *B. cereus* in boiled and fried rice are described in Chapter 6.

Cake mixes

Packaged mixtures for cakes and sponges have given rise to many cases and outbreaks of salmonella food poisoning in the USA and Canada due to the inclusion of salmonella-contaminated egg products. It is recommended that such mixes should not be used unless there is assurance either that they do not include egg products, or that those included have been subjected to pasteurization prior to admixture with the other ingredients of the powder.

Salad vegetables and dessert fruit

In large-scale catering it is recommended that vegetables and fruits with thin skins used for salads and dessert should be washed in water containing a solution of sodium hypochlorite. There are opportunities for salmonella contamination from fertilizers and soil as well as from food handlers. To facilitate the correct use of hypochlorite a marked sink should indicate a known volume of water and a small measure used to add the required concentration of solution; 60 to 80 p.p.m. hypochlorite is considered to be satisfactory for this purpose. The household use of hypochlorites for salad vegetables (including watercress) and fruits is also advocated.

The poor sanitary conditions and polluted water in many countries, particularly in the Middle and Far East, emphasize the need for care of vegetables and fruits purchased in shops and local markets. As well as the direct transfer of bacilli and amoebae, causal agents of dysentery, from product to consumer, cross-contamination from raw to cooked vegetables may take place in the kitchen.

PRESERVATION

Most of the methods devised for keeping food safe are concerned with controlling the growth of bacteria and moulds in the food.

Preservatives

As well as heat and cold, chemicals such as salt, nitrite, acid and other preserving substances are used. Permitted preservatives include: sulphur dioxide (50 to 3,000 p.p.m.) which may be added to sausages, minced meat, dehydrated vegetables, dried fruits, various drinks, fruit juice, pulps and syrups, for example; benzoic acid (150 to 2,000 p.p.m.) may be used for soft drinks, fruit and fruit pulp, flavouring syrups and colours, liquid coffee and drinking chocolate; sorbic acid (1,000 p.p.m.) is useful against mould growth in flour confectionery, cheese, marzipan and solutions of food colouring, and it is sometimes included in wrapping papers.

Dehydration, antibiotics and irradiation are also used to kill bacteria or to prevent their growth.

Dehydration

Dehydration to powdered form reduces the moisture content to levels below which micro-organisms cannot grow. This process does not destroy all micro-organisms and the bacterial purity of the product depends on its state of contamination before dehydration. The addition of water will stimulate growth if temperature conditions are suitable and the substance is normally able to support growth.

Antibiotics

The tetracyclines, chlortetracycline and oxytetracycline, were formerly allowed in ice at a concentration of 5 p.p.m. for storage of fish, but future legislation will ban this practice; the presence of antibiotic traces in fish will be illegal. The treatment of whales at the time of killing with chlortetracycline (1 to 2 p.p.m. of the carcass weight) is said to delay decomposition. Antibiotics are not permitted for the preservation of dressed poultry in the USA and they must not be used in ice for the storage of fish nor in water used for spraying fish in the holds of ships. Experiments showed that when spoilage flora was repressed by chlortetracycline a strain of *S. typhimurium* resistant to the antibiotic grew more readily on dressed broiler chickens that were fed with the organism during life.

The proportion of antibiotic-resistant strains of *S. typhimurium* rose sharply when antibiotics were used freely in animal feeds and for prophylactic measures as well as for the treatment of animals. Recommendations to limit the use of certain antibiotics, except in treatment, to those not normally employed for treating man are given in the Report (Swann) of the Joint Committee on the use of Antibiotics in Animal Husbandry and Veterinary Medicine 1969; they will help to reduce the spread of antibiotic-resistant strains (see Chapter 4, p. 38). Nisin may be used to repress the growth of spoilage organisms in cheese and cream and nystatin is used to prevent mould growth on bananas.

Gamma-rays

Irradiation with small doses of gamma-rays (0·5 to 0·75 Mrad) is recommended for the destruction of salmonellae in foods such as boneless meats, animal feeding meals (bone, fish, meat, cereals) and dried and frozen egg products, for example albumen, where destruction by heat may be difficult.

The use of gamma-irradiation for this purpose has so far been forbidden, but as no harmful effects have been demonstrated and changes in taste and smell are barely detected when small doses of 0·5 Mrad or less are given, it is hoped that the method may come into use and reduce considerably the distribution of salmonellae to animals and man in feeds and foodstuffs.

The hygiene of food storage and preparation depends on a knowledge of the habits of bacteria, the foods they contaminate most frequently, and the temperatures they do and do not like for multiplication. When these facts are known, a common-sense view will enable the more susceptible foods to be protected against the potential danger of contamination with food-poisoning and spoilage bacteria.

SUGGESTED CONDITIONS FOR THE TEMPORARY STORAGE OF FOODSTUFFS

Perishable foods

Certain perishable foods should be kept in a refrigerator maintained at a temperature of 0 to 4·4 °C (32 to 40 °F). These foods include meat, rabbits, game, poultry, fish, shell eggs, milk, cream, fats, butter, lard and margarine. Fish, however, should be kept separately if possible as it readily taints other foods.

Fats, butter, lard and margarine may be kept in a cool room, but if the temperature rises they should be transferred to a refrigerator.

Frosted foods and frozen liquid egg should be kept frozen until required; a temperature of −20·6 °C (−5 °F) is suitable.

Fruit and vegetables should be kept in a cool and well ventilated place protected from frost. Sacks of root vegetables should stand on duck boards to allow the circulation of air.

Dried foods

Dried foods including fruit, fish or meat should be kept in a cool dry place. It is important to avoid conditions which could lead to condensation of moisture on the surface.

RETAIL SHOPS

The number of food-poisoning incidents traced to retail shops is small compared with those reported from hospitals, schools, works and institution canteens, and restaurants including cafés, hotels and holiday camps. One of the reasons for this apparently low proportion is that home incidents are seldom reported and therefore their number is not accurately known. The opportunities for investigation are infrequent and, when they do arise, the responsible food is rarely found; the contaminated food was recognized in approximately 2 per cent of the 546 family outbreaks of salmonellosis occurring in 1968.

Much food will already be contaminated when it reaches the shop and the spread of the organisms will depend on the standard of environmental hygiene, personal cleanliness and storage conditions.

Shops for raw and cooked meats

Each year more than 50 per cent of food-poisoning incidents are traced to contaminated meat and poultry dishes. Some of this illness is caused by the careless handling of cooked products in the home and canteen and also by faulty cooking, cooling and storage methods, but the spread of contamination within the retail shop plays an important role.

Many butchers' shops as well as provision stores sell cooked meats and there is a danger of contamination from raw to cooked meats and between different varieties of cooked meats. In the salmonella outbreak reported on p. 36 it was thought that one infected pig's carcass was responsible for spreading infection to other carcasses in the slaughterhouse where cloths were used to wipe them. More recent work suggests that several pigs were probably infected at the time of slaughter, and that the original infection acquired from contaminated feeding stuffs was distributed over a wide area. The degree of contamination, or the numbers of organisms on a carcass, will depend on various factors but obviously the greater the infection the greater the danger to the retail shop receiving raw meat. In the outbreak quoted several shops selling cooked as well as raw meat were involved. The spread of salmonellae from raw to cooked meat was facilitated by common knives, steels, surfaces, benches, balances and cloths used during the sale of both products. In 1947 few retail shops possessed chilled cabinets and meats of all types were displayed in the windows.

It is doubtful also whether cleaning methods included any form of disinfection and a quick wash-over with cloths would serve to encourage the spread of micro-organisms.

Raw meat should be free from salmonellae but until we have learned how to keep our food animals and poultry free from infection and how to improve the hygiene of slaughter it must be accepted that a variable proportion of the carcasses, boneless meats and sausages sent to retail shops will be contaminated. They should therefore be treated as a potential source of danger to other goods and particularly to prepared meats sold loose from cans and open packs.

The greater the load of bacteria given to cooked meats by the retail shop the shorter their keeping time in the home and canteen

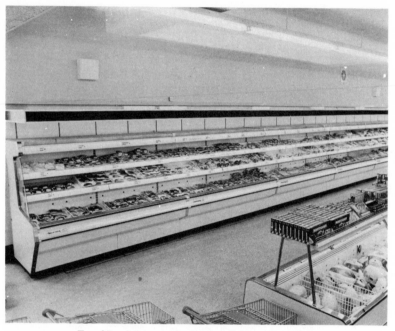

FIG. 25.   Meat products on sale in supermarket

and the greater the danger of the spread of food poisoning organisms and the possibility of food poisoning. The sale of raw and cooked meats should be separated and individual staff, utensils, balances, counters and chill cabinets used for each. In most large shops or supermarkets meat and poultry products are prepacked and sold wrapped (Fig. 25). Care is needed in the sections behind the sales area where these operations are carried out. As in the smaller shops separate utensils and surfaces, used for raw and cooked products, should be cleaned and disinfected frequently in boiling water or chemical agent. Wooden blocks must be scraped and salted daily and where possible replaced by blocks made of impervious material. Five per cent of wood scrapings taken from chopping blocks used in shops for meat were found to contain salmonellae. Hands should be washed frequently and overalls and other apparel often changed.

Wash-hand-basins with running hot and cold water, soap and paper towels should be installed within easy reach of all persons selling not only meat but all perishable foods (Fig. 26). Supplies of boiling water for the disinfection of equipment should be readily

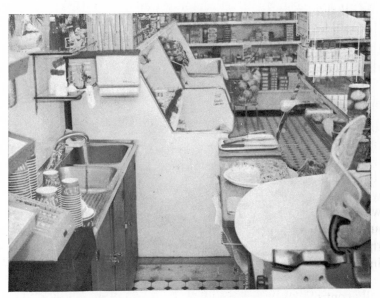

FIG. 26.   Wash-hand-basin in shop near meat display

available; even a gas ring would suffice as a source of heat. The rules for general cleanliness and safety as recommended in the chapters on kitchen design and equipment and the disinfection of utensils also apply to retail shops.

Outbreaks of typhoid fever initiated by meat from cans contaminated by typhoid bacilli during production have emphasized the danger of the spread and persistence of disease-producing organisms in shops where sudden large doses or foci of contamination appear accidentally, and with no visible evidence of their arrival. The management of every shop should question whether the routine cleaning procedures could withstand the spread of infection

from a 2·7 kg (6 lb) block of corned beef contaminated with
S. typhi or other food-poisoning organisms implanted without warning in the shop. Would the cases of illness which must follow the
consumption of this meat be confined to those who purchase parts of
the actual block itself? Or would the bacilli persist on equipment,
spread from meat to meat and to other foods and thus give rise to a
trail of cases for many days? How safe would the staff be under
these circumstances and would those who succumb add to the
spread of infection before diagnosis? Perhaps no one else but the
bacteriologist can visualize the minute trail of bacilli left on the can
opener passing rapidly from can to can, on to the hands and knives
of those who make the first cut and then on to the slicing machine
and other foods; crevices, ledges and cogs are difficult to reach and
they will harbour organisms indefinitely, as will the wide surface of
the cutting blade where fragments of meat caught on the teeth pass
through other blocks of meat sliced on the same machine.

The customer served, the remains of the block may be placed on
one side—or even in the window. The window pedestals, price tags
and trays will all play a part and so also will the sun encouraging a
temperature suitable for multiplication. Overcrowded conditions
will result not only in the jostling of those serving but of the meats
they handle. The hands must be rinsed occasionally and without a
wash-basin nearby a bucket of warm water may be used for hands,
wiping cloths and utensils so that the spread is ensured. Dilute meat
and fat and warmth will encourage survival and growth; if
there is no other way then the water in the bucket must be disinfected.

It is suggested that sliced meat should be prepared under carefully controlled conditions in a room equipped for the purpose at
the rear of the shop, and that the remains of blocks of meat should
be kept refrigerated and separated, as well as the weighed slices.
When the remains of several blocks are gathered into a tray for
refrigeration overnight, the chances of spread from portion to
portion will be increased.

Toilet facilities for the staff should be kept clean and maintained
in a good state of repair; bactericidal soaps and hand creams
may be provided, and nail brushes frequently renewed.

Canned foods ought to be sterile and this is a justifiable assump-
tion by the shop manager so that cool dry storage is adequate.
There are a few notable exceptions. Large cans of ham and pork
shoulder, chopped pork and, more exceptionally, tongue and veal

may receive pasteurization temperatures only; these cans are marked 'keep cold' or 'keep under refrigeration' and it is important to obey this instruction. Organisms which have survived the processing may multiply at atmospheric temperature and spoil the meat, which may also become dangerous. Thus there should be cold storage for stocks.

Open packs, i.e. uncanned, cooked meats and pies, usually leave the factory with a small content of bacteria. If they are exposed in the shop window or on a shelf or bench the numbers of bacteria will increase, the rate depending on the atmospheric temperature and the strength of cure. Thus all such foods should be shown and stored in a chill cabinet maintained at approximately 4 °C (39 °F), until required for immediate sale. The chill cabinet serves many purposes; the food is cold, protected against dust and flies and attractively displayed. Some cabinets have refrigerated shelves or drawers for storage below the display section, others may be combined with a deep freeze.

Various metal gadgets are available to replace the hand for steadying blocks of cooked meats; perforated Perspex covers and plastic plates and blocks are also useful and may easily be cleaned and disinfected.

The sale of vacuum-packed sliced goods increases yearly. Such foods are not sterile and both aerobic and anaerobic bacteria can grow when susceptible foods are stored at atmospheric temperatures; vacuum-packed goods should therefore be kept refrigerated. They should be coded with the date of manufacture and a careful rotation of packs maintained.

After packing some sliced meats are scalded, and hams and large cuts of bacon may be plunged into boiling water to shrink the polythene bag into close contact with the surface. Heat-sensitive surface organisms are destroyed and the storage life is lengthened.

With highly salted goods, such as bacon, growth of many bacteria will be slow but low salt meats of normal pH will encourage microbial growth. When refrigeration arrangements failed for a large batch of film-packed hams delivered to various shops there was a widespread outbreak of staphylococcal food poisoning.

The domestic consumer may consider vacuum packs akin to canned goods and tend to store them in the larder for indefinite periods of time. Some manufacturers give code numbers with expiry dates and recommendations; others give no instructions whatsoever.

The fish shop

There are two recommendations for the fish shop—the closure of shop-fronts and the installation of refrigerated slabs and show cases (Fig. 27).

All open-fronted shops, whether used for the sale of fish or of other foods, are subject to many sources of contamination from the air, passers-by, animals and insects; furthermore, there seems no good reason why the smell of fish should so readily pervade the street. It is true that the closed shop must be well ventilated to

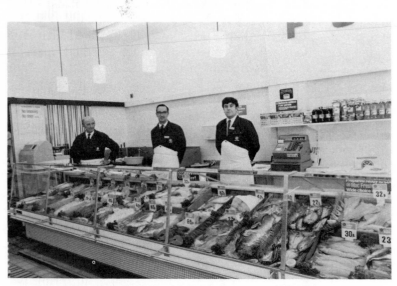

FIG. 27.   Refrigerated slab and showcase of fish shop

prevent the same nuisance to employees. Most fish reach the shop already cleaned and deheaded; nevertheless a small amount of gutting and filleting is inevitable and a separate room or compartment at the back of the shop should be provided for this purpose. It has been shown that fillets of fish, because they have been much handled, are far more likely to contain food-poisoning bacteria of human origin than whole fish. There should be ample supplies of water and facilities for washing the hands, fish and equipment.

It has already been noted (p. 61) that food poisoning from freshly cooked fish is uncommon, but when precooked or left-over fish is mixed with cooked potato, rice or other material for pies, rissoles, and kedgeree, food-poisoning bacteria may be introduced and multiply.

Cooked shell-fish are subject to the same hazards of handling and cockles may be contaminated at many points after their heat treatment in the cockle sheds and before they reach the consumer. Cockles for distribution to far distant places are heavily salted; those for local distribution are lightly salted only and more susceptible to contamination.

A greater use could be made of crushed ice in fish shops. On refrigerated counters or in refrigerated showcases the fish may rest or be embedded in the ice. Regulations for the manufacture of ice have recently been considered.

The organism *Vibrio parahaemolyticus* is associated in the Far East with food poisoning from seafoods eaten raw or cooked. A recent episode of food poisoning amongst passengers landing in London after a flight from Thailand was caused by *V. parahaemolyticus* in hors-d'oeuvre containing crab cooked in the eastern flight kitchen. The outbreak is described in detail in Chapter 6.

V. parahaemolyticus has also been isolated from samples of frozen cooked prawns imported from Malaysia, and in retrospect certain outbreaks of food poisoning may have been associated with prawn cocktails. There are reports that *V. parahaemolyticus* has been isolated from coastal waters and sea creatures in various parts of the world including England. Care should be taken in the sale of crab, shrimps, prawns and fish. They should be stored and exhibited in the chilled state, and care in handling and separation from other foods are important factors.

Grocery and provision stores

Most articles for sale in small provision stores are canned, packaged or otherwise wrapped and therefore protected from contamination. Fats such as lard, margarine and butter may act as vehicles of infection for enteric illnesses and dysentery which may follow infection by small doses of organisms, but they do not usually allow multiplication of the common food-poisoning organisms. Nevertheless, an outbreak of staphylococcal food poisoning was reported from butter sauce. Matured hard cheese has too low a moisture content to allow multiplication, but bacteria can grow when the curd is forming during manufacture. Soft non-acid cheese should be covered and kept cold.

The large provision store or supermarket selling most foods as

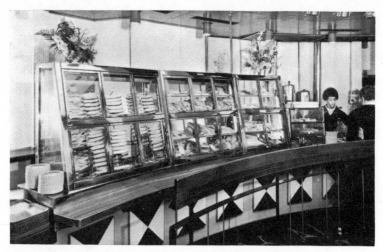

FIG. 28.   Glass cabinets in railway buffet

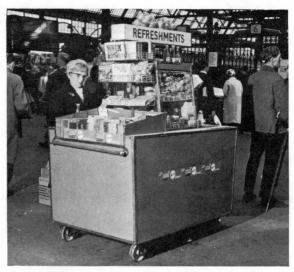

FIG. 29.   Trolley at railway station

well as hardware goods is rapidly crowding out the small shop. Faults in technique will be magnified in their results because food is handled on a large scale and there are increased numbers of customers. Moreover there is a diversity of meats sold in large quantities. A single batch could spread contamination to other meats by a variety of means such as the slicing machine, knives and other equipment, surfaces and hands, so that the number of persons infected could far exceed those who consumed the original contaminated article. Conversely the provision of good practices of cold storage and cleaning procedures will safeguard the health of large numbers of people. Meat slicers and other equipment should be easily and frequently dismantled, cleaned thoroughly and subjected to heat or chemical treatment to destroy as many organisms as possible. Convenient and adequate hand-washing facilities and disposable paper swabs should be provided.

Perishable foods ought not to be exhibited in the window unless chilled, and again it is important to separate raw and cooked meat products. Surfaces should be easily cleaned.

The baker's shop

The preparation and service of confectionery containing fresh or imitation cream requires the greatest care and attention. Manufactured, pasteurized imitation cream may reach the bakery in a state of bacterial cleanliness but there are many opportunities for contamination in the bakery or shop. Such goods should be stored covered under chilled conditions and for a limited time. Commodities which are not wrapped should be handled with tongs and not with the fingers.

Bread is rarely a vehicle of food poisoning because it has a low moisture content and does not encourage bacterial growth. Nevertheless, the bacteria causing typhoid fever and dysentery in small doses may be transported from the hands of an excreter via bread to the victim; bread should therefore be wrapped. Moulds grow well on bread and particularly on sliced bread wrapped while still warm. Although they do not appear to give rise to gastroenteritis there is another serious hazard. Some fungi growing on or within foods are known to produce toxins; the most well known is aflatoxin, from *Aspergillus flavus*, which causes liver disease when fed in mouldy ground-nuts to poultry and fish. Evidence of harmful effects in man is slow to come but it is suggested that more attention should be given to acute or chronic illness in persons accidentally eating mouldy food and in peoples of nations habitually consuming fungi as food or in food.

Bakeries may play an important rôle in the spread of infection from contaminated egg products, meats, coconut and creams. Equipment such as mixers, bowls, working surfaces and Savoy bags should be frequently sterilized. Batches of cream, meats or rehydrated products left over from each day's supply should be discarded or refrigerated for one night only; they should not be mixed with freshly made-up batches. Care should be taken that egg mixes or other products used for glazing are known to be free from salmonellae. The premises should be kept free from dust to which they will be prone because of the flour and other powdered products used.

The dairy

The responsibility for the hygiene of milk is largely the concern of those engaged in pasteurization and bottling. Many dairy shops sell a variety of other foods including ice-cream.

There are no Regulations governing the hygienic quality of fresh cream; most supplies are made from pasteurized milk or they are heat treated as cream, but many are still poor bacteriologically, and need stricter control with regard to both preparation and storage.

Buffets and markets

Perishable foods displayed at buffets on stations, airports, fairs, street markets and in mobile vans should be protected against dust, flies, airborne droplets and animals. Sandwiches, pies, cakes, rolls and similar foods should be wrapped in Cellophane or stand under glass covers or on shelves protected from the air on three sides. They should be freshly prepared and stored for a limited time only.

In many modern glass cabinets the foods, packaged or prepared on plates, are accessible to the customer through glass flaps in the compartments (Fig. 28). Small trolleys pushed around railway platforms are now covered in and the food protected with Cellophane (Fig. 29).

12
Cleaning Methods

Food may be contaminated from dirty utensils, surfaces and equipment; pathogenic organisms may be left in food particles or moisture on imperfectly washed crockery and utensils. The word 'dirty' implies not only the presence of visible dirt but also the invisible presence of thousands and even millions of bacteria which might infect people and contaminate foodstuffs.

It is unsafe to use contaminated utensils and containers, particularly for cooked foods not intended for immediate consumption.

DISH-WASHING

Dish-washing is considered by some to be an unpleasant and tedious occupation, and the work is too often poorly paid. Yet the task is important both aesthetically in the presentation of appetizing food and the appearance of table equipment, and to safeguard health.

The methods in general use for cleaning cooking and eating utensils may be divided into two groups: hand-washing and machine-washing. Both these systems should start with the removal of left-over food, followed by a preliminary rinsing in hot water, to preserve the cleanliness of the wash water.

Hand dish-washing

The laboratory examination of crockery and cutlery, washed in one sink or bowl and immediately wiped without rinsing, has shown that large numbers of bacteria are still present. When a final rinse is given, either in a bowl of hot water distinct from the wash water or by means of running hot water, the results are much improved and the articles may be almost sterile. Running hot water supplied by a boiler system or a water heater is not always available, but a bowl of hot rinse water is practicable for everyone.

When there is a lack of facilities a detergent with bactericidal properties for the wash water or a disinfectant added to the rinse water is recommended.

Two-sink system

When two adjacent sinks are available the first should be used for washing in water with soap or other detergent as hot as the hands can bear, 46 to 50 °C (115 to 122 °F); the second sink should be used for rinsing with very hot water, and methods are available for maintaining high temperatures. The simplest and one of the most effective methods to cleanse and disinfect crockery and cutlery is the two-sink system which provides an efficient wash in a good detergent followed by rinse water thermostatically controlled at a temperature of 77 to 82 °C (170 to 180 °F). Galvanized iron or stainless steel sinks heated by steam, gas or electricity may be used but the greatest uniformity of heat is provided by electricity. A thermometer should be placed in an obvious position on the sink so that the staff will be able to see it easily. Such units require little space, they are relatively inexpensive and they are popular in

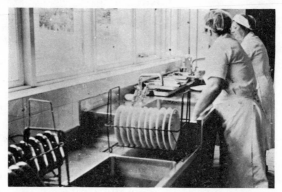

FIG. 30.   Twin-sink heat disinfection unit in a school kitchen

school canteen kitchens, as well as in the kitchens of catering firms (Fig. 30).

The hot rinse not only rids plates, glasses and utensils of wash water, cleaning agents, and bacteria, but it also allows them to drain and dry quickly without the use of drying cloths, which may serve to recontaminate the articles with bacteria. Wash and rinse waters should not be continually used when they have cooled, for lukewarm water will encourage the survival and multiplication of bacteria introduced from food particles. Drying cloths used to wipe a series of articles from such waters will become charged with bacteria—sometimes of intestinal origin (Fig. 31). Laboratory experiments have shown that bacteria from contaminated drying cloths may spread from plate to plate.

There is danger, also, from plates stacked while wet with dirty wash or rinse water. The surface of clean, dry crockery will not encourage the survival of bacteria, whereas microbes left in pools or films of water not only survive but multiply. It is desirable, therefore, that crockery should be left clean, dry, and ready for the next meal; plates taken from hot water should be left to drain vertically in a rack. It has been proved that utensils artificially contaminated with non-sporing bacteria can be disinfected by exposure to hot water at 77 to 82 °C (170 to 180 °F) for approximately 30 seconds and that china and utensils rinsed with water maintained at this temperature will dry rapidly in the air.

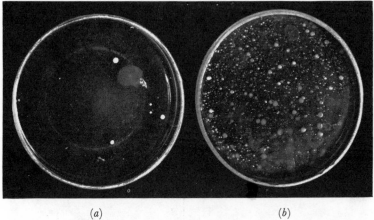

(a)   (b)

FIG. 31.   Bacterial cultures from (a) a clean and (b) a dirty drying cloth

Disposable paper may be used for final drying and polishing (Fig. 32a); but when it is considered necessary to use cloths they should be washed and boiled frequently, or washed and treated with hypochlorite or other bactericidal agent (Fig. 32b).

There is another two-sink system made of stainless steel whereby hot water from a gas boiler flows continuously to the rinse sink, rinse water circulates into the wash sink containing a cleansing agent, and the wash water flows away. Thus it is impossible for food waste to accumulate either in the wash or in the rinse water.

Most materials used for containers and other articles of equipment, can withstand hot water and those which cannot should not be used for foods.

Chemical disinfection

Heat is recommended as the safest method to ensure the destruction of micro-organisms, but it may be impossible to maintain a continuous supply of nearly boiling water or steam. Treatment in rinse water containing chlorine or in wash water containing a bactericidal detergent are the alternatives. The quantity of detergent used should be carefully controlled; too much may affect the flavour and odour of foods, too little will be ineffective; there may be no means of observing when the disinfecting action has been exhausted. The worker cannot assess the rate of decline in efficiency of chemical disinfection; therefore, the instructions given by the manufacturer must be followed carefully, and the correct quantities of substances added to a known volume of water.

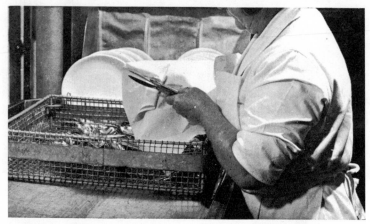

FIG. 32(a).   Disposable absorbent paper used for final drying and polishing

Hypochlorite and quaternary ammonium compounds are used most commonly but other chemicals are available.

Hypochlorites are readily destroyed by food debris and by very hot water. Some are destructive to silverware and stainless steel, and they may be harmful to cloth.

The names of bactericidal substances recommended by the dairy industry are given in a list of approved chemical agents issued by the Ministry of Agriculture, Fisheries and Food.

Until another list is formulated for the food industry there seems no reason why guidance should not be sought from dairy usage.

To assist in hand-washing crockery and utensils a mop with a plastic frame and Nylon bristles is recommended; it should be well cleaned and disinfected overnight in a suitable chemical solution.

Cloths for wet-mopping and cleaning should not be used in the kitchen; disposable paper is recommended to replace them (Fig. 32c).

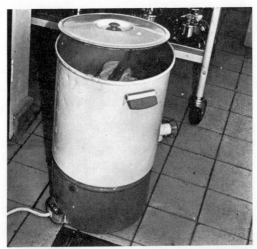

FIG. 32(b).   Disinfecting cloths by boiling

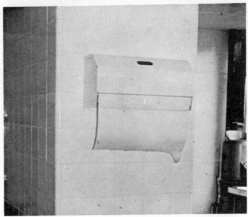

FIG. 32(c).   Disposable paper and holder

In some countries the disinfection by heat of all eating, drinking and cooking utensils is compulsory. Where there is no special apparatus to ensure adequate heat treatment, common receptacles such as bowls and saucepans are used. The containers may be placed on a perforated disk over boiling water heated on a gas ring or other convenient source of heat.

Machine dish-washing

Machines for dish-washing are used in many large-scale catering establishments. Most designs include detergent and rinse sprays, the temperatures of which can be controlled and maintained at 49 to 60 °C (120 to 140 °F) and 66 to 82 °C (150 to 180 °F) respectively (Fig 33). A hand- or foot-operated spray may be installed for removing gross particles of food from plates and other articles before they are stacked. The plates are stacked in carrier racks, so that their maximum surface is exposed to the jets of water which play over them from above and below as the racks pass through the

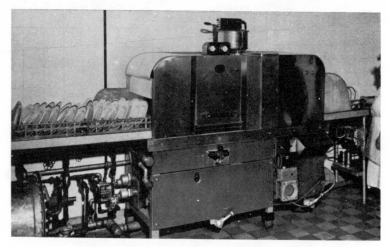

Fig. 33.   Large spray-type dish-washing machine

machine on a movable belt. The whole process is short and takes no longer than 40 to 45 seconds.

The wash water, containing a suitable detergent, is held in a tank and is continually re-used; the overflow runs away to waste. The concentration of detergent must be reinforced from time to time. Some machines include a gadget for automatically dispensing the detergent at regular intervals. The rinse water comes straight from the mains and is usually recirculated into the wash tank. On the more elaborate machines there may be a final row of sprays delivering mains cold water; this water is not recirculated but runs to waste. Usually the articles are delivered hot and steaming from the machine and they are rapidly air-dried.

The efficiency of cleaning and disinfection by these machines depends largely on the maintenance of the wash and rinse waters at the correct temperatures and on the use of a good detergent at the recommended concentration. A machine used carelessly may give bacteriological results no better than those from the worst type of hand-washing.

In one establishment operatives were observed to be wiping the plates emerging after treatment in a newly installed machine. They explained that there were food particles on the plates; several faults were found. The plates were badly stacked on the racks, the detergent was unsuitable because it produced excessive amounts of froth and the temperature of the rinse water was too low. The results obtained from the examination of plate swabs gave very high bacterial counts, the highest noted for machine-washed articles. In another large washing machine the metal runway which should have drained the water from the exit end of the machine to the sink did not slope sufficiently to allow the water to run away. Pools collected, and the examination of this water showed that it contained many millions of bacteria. The plates were stacked in piles of 6 to 12 on the runway so that the bottom plate of each pile became heavily contaminated with bacteria, which were passed on to a second plate when one pile was added to another.

There are smaller spray-type machines that can be worked by one operative, in which wash and rinse sprays are contained in one unit (Fig. 34). The articles are placed in racks which are lifted by hand into the machine. A manually operated lever controls the flow of the wash and rinse waters from the upper and lower sprays. The timing is not automatically controlled, and therefore each operative must judge the length of time articles should be exposed to the wash and rinse waters.

The less complicated types of dish-washing machines include two- and three-tank systems employing brush or turbulent (Fig. 35) mechanisms for the forceful removal of food particles. The brushes have Nylon bristles, which are cleaned more easily than pig bristles; these machines have heating elements to provide the correct temperatures for wash and rinse waters. Small units with two or three sinks may be seen in school canteens, as well as in restaurant kitchens. Wash and rinse waters are maintained at nearly boiling point and the wash tank is supplied with a propeller which continually churns the water. Racks containing the dishes and cutlery are placed in the wash and rinse sections for a convenient length of time. The method is probably too slow for establishments using a large number of plates at any one time, but the bacteriological results from articles washed in this way are good.

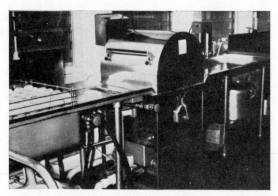

FIG. 34.   One-man-operated small domestic dish-washer

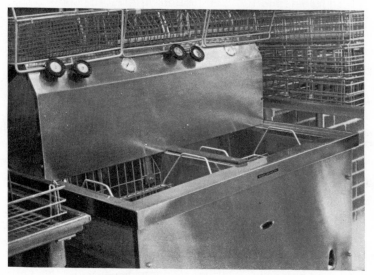

FIG. 35.   Two-sink, turbulent dish-washer

The method shown in Fig. 36 eliminates the stacking of used tableware in the dining area. The self-service trays are flowed directly on the conveyor by the diner and dealt with by the machine operators who are engaged for the purpose. The machine used gives four separate washes, rinse, wash, heated rinse, and high-powered heated rinse.

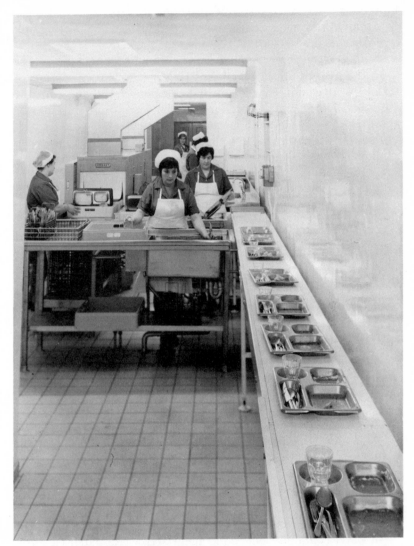

FIG. 36.   Machine washing of self-service trays

In a survey of 20 restaurants and canteens the main divisions for classification were based on washing-up methods, and efficiency was judged by bacterial counts. The classification was carried out as follows:

1. Premises with one sink only.

2. Premises with twin sinks—wash-rinse arrangements.
3. Premises having two sinks—the second being a disinfecting sink maintained at a constant temperature.
4. Premises using a mechanical dish-washing machine.

In the first group, in which one sink only was used, 28 lots of articles were examined, such as plates, spoons, forks, and cups; 14 of these showed contamination with bacteria from the nose or throat, and 9 of them with intestinal bacteria.

In group two, the general bacteriological standard showed a slight improvement over that in the first group, but high counts, sometimes in the region of some thousands per utensil, were obtained. Thirty-one lots of articles were examined; 4 showed contamination with organisms from the nose and throat, and 6 with intestinal organisms.

In the third group, giving the best results, long-handled metal racks were used for the immersion of crockery and utensils for not less than 30 seconds in a disinfecting rinse sink maintained at a temperature of 77 to 82 °C (170 to 180 °F). Thirty-eight lots of articles were examined; 3 only showed contamination with nose and throat organisms and 3 showed contamination with organisms from the intestine. Plates were not wiped, but stored in the hotplate containers; cutlery, however, was wiped to prevent rusting. At least 53 per cent of articles in this group attained the United States Public Health standard of 100 or less bacteria per utensil and absence of any respiratory and intestinal organisms.

The results for group four, using machine methods of dish-washing, varied widely according to the type of machine and the care with which it was run. The temperatures of the rinse waters from most of the machines were far below those recommended, and in many instances the utensils were hand-dried as they were taken out. In this fourth group the best results were obtained from a twin-sink machine, already described, fitted with a thermostatically controlled heating mechanism in both wash and rinse sinks. The wash water contained a cleaning agent and was agitated violently by means of a paddle, and water in the heated rinse tank was maintained at a temperature of about 82 °C (180 °F). In some models of this machine a third tank is included in which the crockery and utensils are freed from cleaning agents before they are transferred to the disinfecting rinse. All tank waters were changed at intervals of 2 hours. Swabs taken from crockery and utensils were bacteriologically sterile.

The unsatisfactory results obtained from some machines were obviously due to lack of care in the supervision and running of machines. Thirty-five lots of articles were examined in this group; of these, 15 showed contamination with organisms of respiratory origin and 11 with organisms of intestinal origin.

A certain number of kitchens were visited daily for a week or more; the counts obtained from the samples taken each day varied

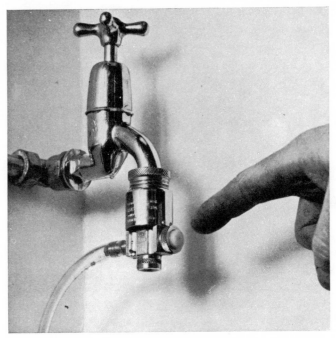

FIG. 37. Detergent dispenser

considerably. Sometimes the variation was associated with a change of technique. For instance, damp cloths were used on some occasions to wipe the plates emerging from the machine, and counts from these plates were high. On other days, when plates were allowed to drain dry without further wiping, counts were much lower.

A few kitchens used a rinse solution containing hypochlorite; the results were regularly good for dishes rinsed in this way. A hypochlorite rinse, if carefully controlled, can produce clean articles almost free from bacteria. It is considered, however, that the routine use of hot-water disinfection is more efficient and practicable for a kitchen staff who may not take time or trouble to control the strength of hypochlorite.

A survey was carried out on six spray-type dish-washing machines used in the staff kitchens of various hospitals. Samples of wash water and swabs of washed articles gave satisfactory bacteriological results because high temperatures were maintained in wash and rinse waters. Experiments showed clearly the importance of high temperatures in both wash and rinse waters for maintaining

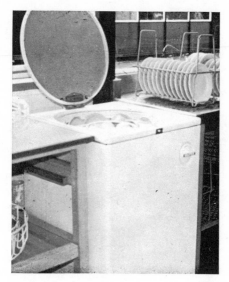

FIG. 38.   Small domestic dish-washer

low bacterial counts. When the temperatures were lowered experimentally the bacteriological results deteriorated and the counts rose in spite of the use of a bactericidal detergent dispensed automatically. A detergent dispenser would help to ensure that crockery and utensils are free from food and grease (Fig. 37). Where circumstances do not permit the use of a steady supply of hot water for washing dishes by hand a bactericidal detergent or another disinfectant agent should be used.

In this survey it was pointed out that a pre-rinse was desirable so that food debris would be removed and the wash water kept cleaner; this is applicable to both hand- and machine-washing of dishes.

Racks and baskets specially designed for the size and type of crockery and to hold cutlery upright were recommended.

The small domestic dish-washer (Fig. 38) is useful for the large household or small canteen. The ease of stacking, the provision of a final hot rinse, and in addition steam, followed by time for articles to drain dry are essential considerations.

The visual criterion of efficiency is a clean plate or utensil, but a test in which fine powder, as used for finger prints, is puffed on to plates and sticks to areas which are not clean has proved to be of value.

Pot washing

It is equally important to have proper facilities to clean pots, pans and other vessels and utensils used in the preparation of food. The large tanks so frequently designed for the purpose seem built for persons of giant proportions; their depth and width require reaching and bending guaranteed to cause backache and strained limbs. Furthermore, a considerable volume of water is required to fill them and, once filled, the same water may remain throughout the whole operation. Samples of water from these tanks give very high counts of intestinal bacteria. The installation of machines for pot-washing relieves congestion and gives rise to a higher standard of cleanliness. The King Edward Hospital Fund for London have issued a report describing the efficiency of a mechanical pot-washer installed in the kitchen of a hospital supplying nearly 2,000 meals daily.

A final rinse in very hot water is equally important for pots, pans and utensils used for preparation and cooking, and they should be air-dried.

Detergents

A detergent is a cleaning agent made of soap or a soap substitute; it may be a mixture of alkaline materials and a substance which will soften the water, or it may be an organic surface-active agent. Its function in dish-washing is to facilitate the removal of food particles from the dishes and utensils and promote cleanliness so that all surfaces are readily accessible to the disinfectant action of heat or chemicals.

The selection of a detergent for a particular purpose will depend on certain factors, such as the nature of the substance to be removed, the material of the article or the surface to be cleaned, whether the hands must come in contact with the solution or whether it will be used in a machine, and the chemical nature of the water such as its degree of hardness. It may be an advantage to use a cleaning agent possessing some bactericidal power. Recommendations for the use of any type of detergent will depend on the particular set of circumstances.

The majority of detergents are cleansing agents possessing little or no bactericidal properties, but some organic substances, such as the quaternary ammonium compounds, are able to kill certain bacteria. Other detergents may combine good cleansing substances with a hypochlorite, so that the two functions of cleaning and disinfection may be accomplished by the one liquid or powder. Such mixtures may be used in small establishments with limited washing-up facilities, such as country cottages, the small kitchen attached to a hospital ward, and the fair or sports ground, and for the bacterial cleanliness of ice-cream servers, cups, and other utensils used by mobile vans. They may be used also by the food vendors for washing their hands.

The general properties of a good detergent should include:

1. Wetting—the ability to wet readily the utensils being cleaned.
2. Emulsification—the ability to break up and disperse fat.
3. Dissolving—the ability to dissolve food materials, principally protein.
4. The ability to break up any solid food matter, no matter what it is.
5. The prevention of scum and scale formation in hard water.
6. Rinsing—the property of being easily rinsed away.
7. Harmlessness to man.

No one substance possesses all the required properties, and most proprietary detergents contain a mixture of ingredients but the exact formulae are seldom divulged.

Soap is a simple detergent, but its use for washing-up is limited in hard water. It is well known that in hard water the washing of greasy dishes with soap results in scum formation. This scum is a mixture of dirt and hard magnesium and calcium salts from the water which have been precipitated out of solution by the soap. A water softener is an agent which keeps the salts of hard water in solution so that the cleaning agent itself may be more effective.

Most good detergents incorporate a water-softening agent.

Some substances used for this purpose are common washing soda (sodium carbonate), trisodium phosphate and sodium metasilicate and also the hexametaphosphate, tetraphosphate and pyrophosphate salts of sodium.

Sodium hydroxide is a good dissolving agent but its caustic action is injurious to the skin. A good inorganic detergent powder may contain a mixture of sodium hydroxide or sodium carbonate, trisodium phosphate, sodium metasilicate, and sodium hexametaphosphate, thus combining cleansing and water-softening properties. The proportion of each ingredient must depend on the purpose for which the powder is intended and the hardness of the local water. These strongly alkaline powders are useful for many purposes, such as for crockery, cutlery, and milk, ice-cream or other food containers. It must be remembered that they are hard on the hands and, therefore, best used in machine-washing where a cleaning agent which does not froth is of particular value.

The organic detergents include those which are manufactured as a by-product of the oil industry. Many are negatively charged (anionic) and can be used in combination with soap, which is also anionic. They possess most of the properties which make a good detergent; they wet readily, emulsify fats, break up dirt particles, and soften the water by keeping calcium and magnesium salts in solution. They are not usually alkaline and are preferable to the caustic inorganic powders for hand-washing. On the other hand they often froth too much to be of value in dish-washing machines. The anionic detergents are sometimes mixed with a hypochlorite to combine cleaning and disinfecting properties. The quaternary ammonium compounds are cationic detergents, that is, they are positively charged and cannot be mixed with soap. Some foam readily while others do not. They exert a bactericidal action on some germs and may be mixed with inorganic materials to form satisfactory cleaning and bactericidal agents.

There is another group of organic detergents, or surface-active agents as they are called, which are non-ionic—that is, they have neither a negative nor a positive charge. They have good wetting properties in cold water and are useful detergents with good stability towards hard water, acids and alkalis.

All articles should be rinsed free from cleaning agents as it is not always known whether harmful effects could arise from the accumulation within the body of small doses of some of the wide range of substances used.

The washing of glassware in licensed premises

The conditions which prevail for washing glasses in licensed premises are different from those for dish-washing in other catering establishments. All cleaning is done at the bar counter, and at rush hours there is a considerable turn-over of glasses in a short time. It is necessary, therefore, that some system should be designed for quick washing and for the disinfection of these glasses.

An island should be provided behind the bar where all glasses and other drinking utensils are washed either by the bar attendant or by staff specially engaged for washing-up duties. The two-sink procedure should be used, and it is recommended that an adequate supply of glasses should be available, to allow time for the washed glasses to cool before they are required for further use. Cloth-drying after a hot rinse would be unnecessary, but to impart a final polish to the glasses a clean dry cloth or paper could be used on the dry glass.

In places where it would be difficult to install two tanks it is suggested that a combined chemical agent and detergent should be used in the single tank, but there must be properly controlled use of the bactericidal substance combined with sufficient changes of water in the tank, and the adequate supply and use of clean dry cloths or paper.

A bactericidal detergent, such as a quaternary ammonium compound, added to the water used for washing beer glasses reduces the number of residual bacteria on the glasses. It is recommended that an automatic dispenser (Fig. 39) be used to deliver a constant dose of the cleaning and disinfecting agent into a sink of known capacity. A quick rinse in a bowl of tepid water should not be tolerated.

Special small washing machines for glasses are available which can be fixed to the bar itself. Used glasses are subjected to a detergent wash and a hot rinse spray; if it is desired to cool the glasses rapidly, a cold spray can be used finally (Fig. 40). Although it is recommended that machine-washed glasses should be air-dried or used wet, there are conventional objections to these procedures; clean, dry cloths or paper should therefore be available.

The large food container and other equipment

Amongst the more important articles to be kept clean and free from bacteria are the large food containers used to transport meals from central school kitchens to the children in surrounding schools and also those used for carrying food from the kitchen to the

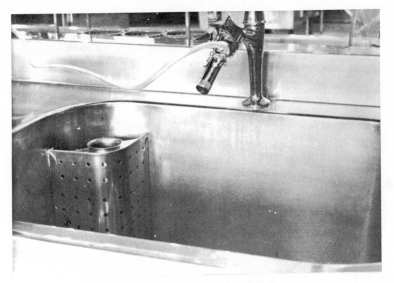

Fig. 39. Detergent dispenser for public house

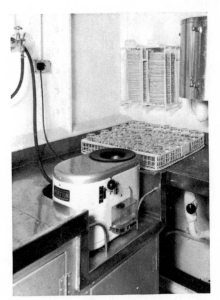

Fig. 40. Glass-washing machine

wards of hospitals. There should be provision for the disinfection of these containers and for their subsequent drainage. Food residues, if allowed to remain, may retain bacteria able to contaminate the next batch of food.

When freed from all residual food particles, each container should be thoroughly washed in a warm detergent solution, rinsed free from the wash water, steam heated and drained; the inside should not be touched again before it receives the freshly prepared food. It has been shown that high bacterial counts are common from containers washed in the ordinary way and cloth-dried. Cooked food may remain in these containers for a considerable time, and it is necessary to ensure that bacteria which remain on the inner walls in spite of thorough cleaning are destroyed by steam and that more bacteria are not introduced by contaminated cloths. The lids of the containers should also be steamed.

The time of exposure to steam, from a jet or in a cabinet or in a machine, should be adequate. Immersion in tanks of boiling water may also be used.

As an alternative measure, where there are no facilities for treatment with steam, a final rinse in hypochlorite solution should be given.

It is not intended here to give detailed information on the cleansing of plant equipment used in food manufacture; it is necessary only to stress its importance. This is particularly true for ice-cream equipment, the cleanliness and sterility of which is essential for the purity of the ice-cream mix and for the maintenance of Grade I samples. It is probable that the same applies to many other foodstuffs manufactured with the help of machines.

The basic principles of any cleansing technique include a hot detergent wash, followed by some method of disinfection by water, which should be nearly boiling, steam or chemical agent. Hand cloths to dry equipment should be used only when hot water is unobtainable and chemical disinfection is used; the drying cloths should be washed and boiled frequently or paper used. Preferably, articles should be air-dried rapidly, or absorbent paper may be used, and stored dry.

Infant feeding bottles and other food containers

Infants and young children are very susceptible to intestinal infections and the proper care of feeding bottles and teats is an important factor in preventing the spread of enteritis amongst infants.

The Medical Research Council Memorandum No. 11 (Revised Edition 1951) recommended that, when feeds are finished, the bottles should be thoroughly rinsed in cold running water, cleansed with a detergent to remove milk film and rinsed again in running water. Brushes used for cleansing bottles should be disinfected after each period of use. Teats and valves should be turned inside out after each use, gently scrubbed to remove all traces of feed, and boiled for not less than 2 minutes before being used again. Between each feed, bottles should be disinfected by boiling for not less than 2 minutes in special equipment. Chemical disinfection with a hypochlorite solution may be used also. The results compared with those from the boiling method showed that sterility could generally be obtained by the use of either hypochlorite or heat provided the correct technique was used; care is needed to submerge teats.

When milk feeds for infants are prepared in bulk, terminal sterilization of the assembled feed in the bottle is the safest method. The prepared feed is boiled and added to sterilized bottles; then the sterilized teats are affixed and capped and the whole unit is sterilized by steam under pressure in an autoclave or pressure cooker.

Food containers for infant food

All containers and utensils used for broths and purees fed to infants during the second 6 months of life should be disinfected in boiling water and drained dry without wiping.

CLEANING PREMISES AND EQUIPMENT

Daily cleaning should remove all traces of the day's activities; food scraps and smears should be removed and working benches should be washed over with hot water and detergent; meat and poultry sections should be finished with a disinfectant agent and mopped up with disposable paper rather than cloths.

Fish slabs should be scrubbed down with hot water, detergent and bactericidal agents; meat blocks should be scraped, and rubbed over with salt, scrubbed with detergent and wiped over with a cloth wrung out in hypochlorite solution. Sweeping and dusting should be done with damp cloths and dust-damping powders. Floor surfaces most suitable for kitchens should withstand scrubbing with hot, soapy or detergent water. Fixed carpets and mats should be vacuum-cleaned daily. At weekly intervals service pipes and exposed framework of roof or ceiling, light bulbs and shades, and floor-draining channels should be washed or dusted with a damp cloth. A vacuum cleaner may be used for overhead fittings as an alternative to damp-dusting.

Articles and equipment with which food comes into contact should be kept clean. Equipment should be designed so as to be readily taken apart and should be so placed that all parts can be easily reached. Disinfection should be applied to equipment used for perishable raw ingredients such as egg products for glazing and for cake, sponge and other flour confectionery mixes, for meats, gelatin, milk and coconut and to all equipment used in the preparation, storage and dispensing of fillings, decorations and toppings.

The general principle of cleaning for all equipment including can openers, meat-slicing machines and mincers should be to pass all disassembled parts through the following stages: hot detergent water, a rinse at 76·7 °C (170 °F) by means of a washing machine or a two-sink system in which the second sink is thermostatically controlled at a temperature of 76·7 °C (170 °F) or higher. When possible there should be a final exposure to steam or immersion in boiling water for about 1 minute. Immovable equipment, covered metal containers and mixers should be exposed to steam from a hose for 10 to 15 minutes. As an alternative to steam or boiling water a chemical disinfectant should be used; probably the most effective are the hypochlorite, iodine or bromine preparations. All surfaces must be thoroughly wetted with the disinfectant, diluted according to the maker's instructions. After a suitable contact period of at least 5 minutes the treated equipment may be rinsed with clean mains water and dried with absorbent paper.

Small articles such as ladles, palette knives and piping bags should be cleaned and boiled or replaced by treated articles after meal breaks.

13

Sterilization and Disinfection

(I. M. MAURER)

The word 'sterilize' is often used incorrectly. Sterilization means the destruction of all micro-organisms of all kinds, including bacterial spores such as those produced by clostridia. Sterilization is not normally necessary in food hygiene. Prevention of the growth of spores is sufficient for the prevention of food poisoning; the spores need not be killed. Unfortunately, the word 'sterilize' is commonly used in the literature of food hygiene and in some official publications where the word 'disinfect' would be correct. Cleaning products are often described as 'detergent/sterilizer' when 'detergent/disinfectant' would be an accurate description. The title 'sterilizing sink' is used although water in a sink cannot be heated above boiling point (100 °C; 212 °F) and the lowest temperature recommended for sterilization is 121 °C (229·8 °F). Most young mothers imagine that they 'sterilize' a baby's bottle when they disinfect it by boiling or chemical treatment. Sterilization of feeding bottles is not necessary although disinfection is required.

In an attempt to clarify the difference between the two words 'sterilization' and 'disinfection' the British Disinfectant Manufacturers Association press release in 1970 defined the words with other related terms. Their definitions are so valuable that they may be repeated here.

Sterilization:	the process of destroying or removing all microbial life.
Disinfection:	the destruction of micro-organisms but not usually bacterial spores; not necessarily killing all micro-organisms but reducing them to a level not normally harmful to health.

A British standard which defines these and similar words is in preparation. It is hoped that its publication will do something to prevent the dissemination of misleading information.

It must be emphasized once again that the word 'sterilize' should be used only for a process which can be depended upon to destroy bacterial spores. Disinfection cannot be depended upon to destroy such spores. They are tough organisms and are difficult to kill. No chemical disinfectant should be described as a sterilizer, or a sterilant.

Disinfection is essential in food hygiene. It may be brought about by:

1. Cleaning.
2. Heat.
3. Chemical disinfectants.

Disinfection by cleaning

Disinfection by cleaning is probably the most useful of the three methods. It may be used alone or in combination with either of the other two. A high proportion of microbial contamination may be removed from premises, equipment and also the hands by thorough cleaning. The standard of cleaning premises and equipment and the level of decontamination achieved depends on several points.

(a) The design, materials and condition of the surfaces and equipment to be cleaned. The design should make it possible to reach all parts with ease and to dismantle equipment, exposing all the soiled areas. Soft and porous surfaces such as plain wood or untreated cork are more difficult to clean than those that are harder and non-porous. Worn, scarred, scratched or chipped surfaces are always difficult to clean.

(b) Individual care and effort affect the level of cleaning more than does the use of a particular cleaning agent. Much depends on the training and supervision of the staff. Failure to change cleaning water when it is dirty will mean failure in decontamination.

(c) Choice of cleaning agents. The wide variety on the market is confusing for the user. No one of them is ideal and more depends on the method by which they are applied than on the choice of a near-perfect agent. In general the costly, fancy cleaning agent of unusual perfume or colour should be avoided as unnecessary. Inexpensive, old-fashioned washing soda is a fine cleaner for greasy equipment, grids over drain-pipes and the pipes themselves. Pouring a washing soda solution into sink waste pipes will do much to keep the sinks unblocked. Scouring powders should not be so harsh that they damage surfaces or eventually cleaning will be impossible. Perfumes are suspect because they hide the bad smells which come from failures in cleaning. Claims for bactericidal action of cleaning agents should be ignored. Many such claims are unsupported by acceptable scientific evidence although the advertising literature may reproduce certificates or seals of approval awarded on grounds which are ill-defined. On some occasions it may be thought advisable to treat kitchen surfaces or equipment with a chemical disinfectant as an extra weapon in the battle against bacterial contamination. Where this is done the maximum benefit is obtained by cleaning first of all and applying the disinfectant afterwards. Combined detergent/disinfectants are of questionable value since they are inevitably applied to a dirty, usually food-soiled, surface. Dirt of many kinds, including scraps of food, inactivates chemical disinfectants. For this reason the use of the chemical disinfectant is always recommended as the second step of a two-step process. Clean first and disinfect afterwards.

(d) Care of the cleaning apparatus, which must itself be kept in a clean hygienic condition, affects cleaning standards. Time is saved by eliminating apparatus where possible. Hot dish-washing means spontaneous drying of crockery and avoids the use of tea towels. Disposable paper towels are hygienic when thrown away after using once. Although this seems to be extravagant there is a saving in labour required to launder linen towels. Disposable cloths for wet work also save labour but, with all disposables, attempts to re-use them must be resisted. Where mops, brushes and cloths are to be used more than once, it will be safer to avoid disposable models and choose varieties which are tough enough to withstand decontamination after use. Cleaning apparatus used for wet work is likely to become heavily contaminated with bacteria unless it is disinfected by heat, or chemicals, as well as being kept clean. In this situation washing mops, cloths and brushes will remove large numbers of bacteria but the few which remain may multiply in a few hours while the apparatus is wet. Next time the apparatus is used it will no longer remove bacteria from soiled surfaces but will increase the bacterial load on the surfaces.

The most effective treatment for wet-cleaning apparatus is heat disinfection combined with the laundering which is described below.

Disinfection by heat

Disinfection by heat is the most reliable of the three methods. Immersion in water at 65 °C (149 °F) for 10 minutes, or at higher temperatures for shorter times, can be depended upon to destroy most micro-organisms harmful to health, with the exception of bacterial spores. For many years it was believed that boiling water could be used to sterilize but now it is known that bacterial spores may survive boiling. However, boiling water is an effective and cheap disinfectant.

Heat disinfection may conveniently be included in a cleaning process. In machine dish-washing, the temperature of the washing or rinsing water may be adjusted and the time arranged to include heat disinfection in the cycle. In manual dish-washing also, this can be arranged in a so-called 'sterilizing' rinsing sink. It would be more accurately described as a disinfecting sink. Here the water is hot enough to disinfect the crockery, and a rinsing temperature of 65 °C (149 °F) or more, will enable it to dry spontaneously and avoid recontamination by unhygienic tea towels.

Similarly, a disinfecting temperature may be included in a laundry cycle, in either the washing or the rinsing process. Heat treatment in laundering will ensure the disinfection of all the tea towels (if they must be used), all dish mops and sponges, floor cloths, damp dusters and floor mops; also the scrubbing brushes used for floors, hands, pans or vegetables. As previously described, all cleaning apparatus used for wet work should be disinfected daily in order to prevent bacterial growth. Heat is not only the most reliable disinfectant, but also the cheapest. A combination of heat disinfection with daily cleansing of the apparatus is hygienic, time saving and economical.

In making up a list of cleaning apparatus needing heat treatment, bowls, buckets and scrubbing machines should not be forgotten, and in all cases materials should be chosen which will withstand the disinfection temperatures. Manufacturers of cleaning equipment are now, in most cases, aware of the need to use materials which will withstand heat. Some new designs for floor scrubbing machines are planned which can be dismantled and heat treated daily to disinfect all parts which become wet.

The practice of applying steam from a hose, in food premises, is a useful method of heat disinfection, although its efficacy is difficult to assess accurately because the conditions are variable. Steam treatment of equipment in a cabinet may also be recommended, but the results are also variable. Times normally quoted for steam disinfection are 5 to 10 minutes' application from a steam hose and 10 to 15 minutes in a steam cabinet.

It must be remembered that bacteria may multiply rapidly in stagnant water. Neglected puddles or wet dregs in food premises, may present a hazard to health. Equipment should always be stored dry and protected from dust during storage.

Disinfection by chemicals

Disinfection by chemicals is widely advertised but is more costly and less reliable than heat disinfection. The effectiveness of chemical disinfection depends on a number of variables which are not always understood.

Some chemical disinfectants are active against a wide range of bacteria but others have a narrow range of antibacterial activity. Staphylococci are among the bacteria which are killed fairly easily by chemical disinfectants. Salmonellae are more difficult to kill by chemicals and the spores of clostridia will usually survive chemical treatment. Some chemical disinfectants are bactericidal, they kill vegetative bacteria but not spores. Others are no more than bacteriostatic, they prevent the growth of vegetative bacteria.

Effectiveness of chemical disinfection depends, to some extent, on the time of contact, the temperature and the concentration of the solution. At least 2 minutes' contact is desirable for the most rapid disinfectant and as long as 30 minutes may be necessary for the effective action of some others. Higher temperatures of disinfectant solutions increase their effectiveness and accurate measurement of the recommended concentration is all-important.

The numbers of bacteria present and their accessibility to a chemical disinfectant must be considered. A few bacteria are more easily killed than many. Those which are hidden by pieces of equipment or under layers of grease may be protected from the chemical action. Dismantling equipment and washing it before exposure to a chemical disinfectant will increase effectiveness.

Many chemical disinfectants will kill some micro-organisms and the best of them will kill a great many, but only if the conditions are favourable. It is unfortunate that many materials which are likely to be present in food premises inactivate chemical disinfectants and by their presence create unfavourable conditions.

A common inactivating material is the hard water which is

found in many districts. All chemical disinfectants perform less well when diluted with hard water than when in distilled water. It is not suggested that distilled water be used for diluting disinfectants but it is worth remembering that some reported results of disinfectant tests refer to dilution in distilled water. A favourable report of the disinfectant's performance in a test may therefore be quite true but unrealistic and a poor guide to the performance which may be expected of the disinfectant in practice.

Chemical disinfectants are inactivated by all kinds of organic material, including food, and the greater the quantity of such material present the greater will be the extent of the inactivation. The advice that equipment be washed first, to remove organic material, and that the disinfectant solution be applied to a clean surface has already been given but it is worth repeating. Large quantities of chemical disinfectants are regularly wasted because they are applied to dirty surfaces. Scraps of food may not only prevent access of the chemical disinfectant to the organisms but may also inactivate the disinfectant. If a chemical disinfectant is to be used at all it is worth while providing it with conditions which will enable it to work well.

Anionic disinfectants such as hypochlorites and phenolics are compatible with anionic or non-ionic detergents but they are inactivated by cationic detergents. Similarly, cationic disinfectants such as quaternary ammonium compounds are compatible with cationic or non-ionic detergents but are inactivated by anionic detergents. Manufacturers of detergents and disinfectants may be consulted on this point. Where a chemical disinfectant rinse is planned to follow a detergent wash it is wise to choose compatible products, otherwise the disinfectant may be inactivated by the detergent which has previously been used to clean the surface. Many other materials have been found to inactivate some chemical disinfectants. These include wood, cork, rubber, cotton, Nylon, cellulose sponge mops and many plastics. It is not unusual to find a disinfectant solution in a bucket of plastic material which inactivates it and which also contains an incompatible detergent which completes the inactivation of the disinfectant and is inactivated in its turn. The solution therefore neither cleans nor disinfects, money is wasted on both detergent and disinfectant, the standard of hygiene is low and food poisoning may result. Elsewhere a chemical disinfectant solution may be used alone, but it may be applied with a mop, cloth, sponge or scrubbing brush made of material which, in its turn, inactivates the disinfectant and renders it ineffective.

Another cause for anxiety is the fact that dilute chemical disinfectant solutions may deteriorate with time. A recommended dilution of a well-chosen chemical disinfectant which is measured accurately into a clean bucket, on a Monday, may be effective in disinfecting surfaces or cleaning cloths soaked in it. However, the same solution allowed to remain in the bucket until the following Friday, may not only be too feeble to disinfect, owing to deterioration, but it may have become a source of infection because bacteria are growing in it.

The best chemical disinfectant, working under the best conditions, will rarely, if ever, kill 100 per cent of the bacteria present. There are likely to be a few survivors, over and above any bacterial spores present. The few survivors are most unlikely to present a hazard unless they have the opportunity to linger in the disinfectant solution for several days as it deteriorates. Under these conditions they may multiply rapidly and become a source of infection. It is therefore of great importance that staff be supervised and, where chemical disinfectants are used, fresh preparation daily be insisted upon, in clean containers. The containers should preferably be not only clean but heat treated as described earlier, to destroy bacteria which may remain in them. It is most unsafe to empty yesterday's disinfectant solution from a bucket, and make up today's new solution in the same wet bucket. The dregs of the old solution will contain a few bacteria at best, and many bacteria at worst. They will have acquired some slight resistance to the particular chemical disinfectant and thus will survive with more than usual ease in the new solution. Where refilling of wet containers continues day after day there may be a carry-over, into the fresh solutions, of bacteria with increasing resistance to the chemical disinfectant, which enables them to multiply rapidly in the solution.

The practice of 'topping up' disinfectant solutions is one which must be sternly condemned.

The correct use of a chemical disinfectant is likely to have more effect on the standard of hygiene achieved in food premises than is its chemical nature, but a brief summary of the properties of the different types available for use in food premises is given here. A few commercial brand names are given for each type. They are examples only and are arranged in alphabetical order, not in order of preference. The list is not exhaustive.

Properties of some different varieties of chemical disinfectants

HYPOCHLORITES are probably the most useful for food premises and they are inexpensive. This group has a wide range of anti-bacterial activity including some activity against bacterial spores which is not shown by other varieties. Hypochlorites have little taste or smell. They are anionic and are incompatible with cationic detergents. The addition of a little (anionic) detergent may be necessary to ensure the wetting of shiny surfaces. Where there is no wetting with the solution there is no disinfection. Hypochlorites are inactivated more easily by organic material than are most other disinfectants; this is their chief disadvantage, but apart from incompatible detergents they show very little inactivation by other materials. Owing to the risk of corrosion, metallic equipment should not be left to soak in a hypochlorite solution.

Examples: Brobat, Chloros, Domestos.

IODOPHORS resemble hypochlorites in antibacterial activity but they are less sporicidal. They are more expensive but are equally acceptable as having little taste or smell. Iodophor disinfectants all incorporate a detergent which may be anionic, non-ionic or cationic. They are considerably inactivated by organic material but show little inactivation by other materials.

Examples: Betadine, Vanodine, Wescodyne.

QUATERNARY AMMONIUM COMPOUND (QAC) disinfectants are popular in some food premises but they have a more limited range of antibacterial activity than hypochlorites and iodophors. They are cationic and are incompatible with anionic detergents but are, in themselves, good detergents. They are considerably inactivated by organic material, by soap, hard water, wood, cotton, Nylon, cellulose sponge mops and a few plastics. Some bacteria grow with ease in QAC solutions and for this reason it is advised that where they are used great care is devoted to the preparation of fresh solutions daily in clean, heat-treated containers.

Examples: Hytox, Nonidet, Shield.

QAC DIGUANIDE mixtures are widely advertised as skin disinfec-tants. They have the disadvantages of the QACs, they are expensive and are not the best choice for food premises.

Examples: Resiguard, Savlon.

PHENOLIC DISINFECTANTS are of several types. The white fluid phenolics and the clear soluble fluids of the lysol type have a wide range of antibacterial activity which is similar to that of hypochlorites and iodophors while being much less easily inactivated by organic material. Their disadvantages lie in inactivation by some plastics and by rubber and, in some brands, a powerful smell. The chloroxylenol phenolic disinfectants show a more narrow range of antibacterial activity and greater inactivation by organic material. Phenolic disinfectants are anionic and they are incompatible with cationic detergents. Some brands incorporate a detergent.

Examples: White fluid phenolics: Izal, White Cyllin.

Clear soluble fluid phenolics: Clearsol, Hycolin, Stericol.

Chloroxylenol phenolics: Dettol.

AMPHOLYTE DISINFECTANTS have a narrow range of antibacterial activity and are readily inactivated by many materials and in particular by hard water, organic matter, wood, rubber, cotton, Nylon, cellulose sponge and plastics. They are good detergents but are costly and they are not recommended as disinfectants.

Example: Tego.

PINE FLUIDS show little disinfectant activity and are not recommended. Many brands are available. All of them have the word 'pine' either incorporated in the brand name or mentioned in the advertising literature.

Those responsible for maintaining a high standard of hygiene in food premises should:

1. Choose heat for disinfection wherever possible.
2. Use a chemical disinfectant when, and only when, the application of heat is impossible.
3. Arrange for equipment and surfaces to be cleaned before disinfection by heat or a chemical solution.
4. Select a chemical disinfectant, where one must be used, from a variety showing a wide range of antibacterial activity. A good choice will be a hypochlorite solution used at a concentration giving 100 to 200 p.p.m. of available chlorine for scrupulously clean surfaces. Slightly lower concentrations are permissible for salads. Where absolute cleanliness cannot be assured, a concentration giving 1,000 or more p.p.m. of available chlorine will be required.
5. Ensure the fresh preparation, daily, of chemical disinfectant solutions, in clean, dry and preferably heat-treated containers.
6. Remember that the effectiveness of a chemical disinfectant depends, very much, on the user.

14

Kitchen Design and Equipment

(The late L. KLUTH)

In the construction of buildings for catering purposes a wide range of structural methods and materials are employed, but the basic requirements for any place to be used for the preparation and service of food must comply with the ordinary standards of stability, durability and protection against the weather which are applicable to all buildings.

It is not appropriate here to describe the many details of construction involved in the erection of buildings; these may be studied at length from textbooks dealing exclusively with the subject. It is sufficient to say that the traditional forms of brickwork, masonry or reinforced concrete with slated or tiled or asphalted roof covering probably cannot be improved upon for permanence; whilst the lighter construction consisting of steel framework covered with corrugated asbestos-cement sheets or filled in with lightweight concrete or hollow blocks is acceptable for buildings where a shorter life is anticipated.

The interior

When it is clear that the building fulfils its primary function as a shelter, the internal arrangements which would be specially suitable for food premises should be considered. For obvious reasons, a kitchen should be on the same storey as and adjoin the dining room. Though the delivery of stores and refuse removal is easier from ground floors or basements, the natural lighting, ventilation and outlook are usually better on upper storeys.

It is generally agreed by those interested in food hygiene that there is less likelihood of food becoming contaminated when the kitchen staff work in congenial surroundings. Certainly it may be assumed that intelligent people made conscious of their responsibilities to the public, and employed in premises where work can be done in an orderly and unhurried manner, can and will pay more attention to the demands of hygiene. Fatigue and strain brought about by cramped conditions, inadequate equipment, a dim light, overwork and noise will predispose to carelessness; while good ventilation and lighting, readily accessible and easily cleaned surfaces make the attainment of sanitary conditions less arduous.

Lay-out

The minimum size of kitchens serving the public, and of certain staff canteens, is, in common with several kinds of other workplace, subject to requirements laid down by the Offices, Shops and Railway Premises Act, 1963. No such room may be so overcrowded as to cause risk of injury to the health of the people working therein, nor may there be less than about 3·7 square metres (40 square feet) of over-all floor area and about 11·3 cubic metres (400 cubic feet) of over-all air space per person. These statutory figures refer to basic room capacity rather than to the space available after allowing for equipment; since kitchen equipment usually occupies a considerable amount of space compared with the number of persons using it, it seems unlikely that there will be many kitchens of 2·4 to 3 metres (8 to 10 feet) high where the standards are not met.

So far as working space is concerned, school kitchens designed and erected by the Department of the Environment and the Department of Education and Science may be taken as a reasonable standard: 1·2 to 1·8 metres (4 to 6 feet) of working and passage distance is allowed between islanded cookers and wall sinks or benches; as a rough guide to floor area of kitchens and other essential accommodation, Table 15, based on post-war school-meals service premises, may be of interest, bearing in mind that midday meals only are prepared.

The British Standard Code of Practice, CP3 (1950) Functional Requirements for Buildings, Chapter VII, Engineering and Utility Services, however, suggests a much more generous scale of kitchen area.

For	100 persons	69·7 sq. metres	750 sq. feet
,,	250 ,,	120·8 ,,	,, 1,300 ,, ,,
,,	500 ,,	232·3 ,,	,, 2,500 ,, ,,
,,	750 ,,	278·7 ,,	,, 3,000 ,, ,,
,,	1,000 ,,	348·4 ,,	,, 3,750 ,, ,,
,,	1,500 ,,	464·5 ,,	,, 5,000 ,, ,,
,,	2,000 ,,	557·4 ,,	,, 6,000 ,, ,,

TABLE 15. Approximate floor areas (in square metres/square feet) of school kitchens

No. of meals	Kitchen	Vegetable store	Dry store	Larder	China store	Boiler house	Staff rooms	Refrigerator capacity (cubic metres/cubic feet)
750 in two sittings	176·5/1,900 including two serveries and wash-up	9·3/100	7·4/80	8·8/96	—*	—†	17·1/184	4·6/50
600 in two sittings	131·9/1,420 including servery and wash-up	9·3/100	7·4/80	6·7/72	—*	—†	13·9/150	2·3/25
500 in two sittings	111·5/1,200 including servery and wash-up	9·3/100	6·7/72	7·4/80	—*	9·3/100	14·9/160	2·3/25
350	69·7/750	8·4/90	8·4/90	6·2/67	4·4/48	6·7/72	6·2/67	1·7/18
250	55·7/600	6·5/70	6·5/70	3·3/36	2·8/30	4·6/50	3·3/36	1·7/18
150	39·0/420	3·3/35	←6·5/70→	←3·8/42→	2·2/24	3·3/36	3·3/35	1·7/18
100	27·9/300	3·3/36	↕	↕	↑	3·3/36	2·8/30	—‡
75	19·5/210	1·5/16	↕	2·6/28	↕	—	—	—‡
40	15·8/170	1·4/15	↕	2·2/24	↕	—	—	—‡

* Provision made elsewhere than in the kitchen
† Hot water supply from main building
‡ Domestic refrigerators included

plus space for cloakroom accommodation, lavatories, rest rooms and manager's office.

The present trend in kitchens is to install preparation equipment at the sides (where waste can be conveniently drained away), and to erect island cooking apparatus in the centre of the room where there can be localized ventilation; but even in the smallest kitchens there is need for division into further compartments for the preparation of different kinds of food prior to cooking, and for washing-up.

Work and production should flow progressively from delivery of goods to storage, preparation and service without return or 'cross traffic'. There are good reasons for siting vegetable storage and preparation nearest the point of delivery in an area well separated from the other parts of the kitchen, to prevent soil from root crops contaminating other foods. The sections for raw meat and raw fish should be well separated from those dealing with cooked and prepared products, including the pastry work, in order to prevent contamination passing from raw to cooked foods. Stores for each department should be adequate.

Floors

Traffic in food rooms may vary from normal foot passage to heavy iron-wheeled trolleys, and the durability of the floor surface must meet the need of the particular premises. Apart from this, the major requirements are that the floor must be impervious to moisture and not adversely affected by grease, salt, vegetable or fruit acids, or other food scraps. The finish of the floor should also be such that joints and crevices should not provide lodging for dirt or for insect pests.

In the construction of the floor, angular corners should be avoided and, in particular, internal angles and the junction of the floor with the skirting should be coved.

Asphalt floors are dust-free and waterproof, and do not provide a harbour for vermin; they are, however, liable to erosion by acids and grease, and they will not bear concentrated weights. Pitch mastic floors, on the other hand, are resistant to damage from the action of fatty acids. Quarry tiles when laid well are excellent in all respects, except that, unless faced with an abrasive material, they are slippery when wet; they can be used for covering whole floors or as a base for free-standing equipment in rooms where the rest of the floor is pitch mastic. This arrangement is probably the most satisfactory.

Soft-wood board and joint floors are to be deprecated since the sub-floor space can provide a harbour for rats and mice; the surface is absorbent and the joints between the boards form dirt pockets and provide refuge for insects. Linoleum, particularly when laid in single or jointless pieces with a mastic adhesive, is an improvement, but it cannot withstand heavy wear or concentrated weight, as may be the case with heavy equipment on feet which have a small sectional area.

Hard-wood blocks or boards are warm and easy on the feet; blocks laid end grain uppermost are best as they do not shrink or warp. While less absorbent than soft wood, they are far from impervious even when well oiled, and they are not entirely suitable in places where there is a likelihood of much waste water reaching the floor.

Plain concrete floors may be dusty and irregular and, when not laid in properly proportioned sections, they may crack and break. The inclusion of granite chips (granolithic) and a proprietary binder, or marble chips (terrazzo) in the cement mix instead of gravel, produces a very fine non-absorbent, pest-proof, and dust-free surface. Terrazzo, however, is slippery when wet and sooner or later cracks appear.

Composition floors are manufactured from a basic cement of magnesium oxychloride and a filler, which may be sawdust, powdered cork, sand or clay, together with a pigment. Many such floors have proprietary names and they are laid by specialist contractors. Neither too much water nor any soap or soda should be used for cleaning them; polish and linseed oil preserve the surface.

Rubber laid as tiles or as strips on adhesive is not recommended for other than domestic kitchens. Although easily cleaned, rot-proof, unattractive to vermin and relatively hard-wearing, it may become dangerously slippery when wet or greasy and may soften and corrode under the influence of fatty acids.

Cork tiles or strips form a pleasant floor finish, easily cleaned and relatively durable. Like rubber, however, they have to be specially laid, and probably cost more than is justifiable for commercial kitchens.

Steel tiles set in cement mortar are extremely useful in situations where there is heavy traffic.

Plastic tiles, especially well laid asbestos-vinyl tiles, appear to have properties of equal value to those of quarry tiles.

The main objective at all times should be that the floor be impervious, easily cleaned and durable.

Walls

Unfortunately there does not seem to be a wall finish which will satisfy the two major requirements for food rooms in which there is steam. Walls must be smooth and impervious, to allow easy cleaning, but it is also desirable that the surface should be warm and of an open texture to minimize condensation. Until a material which combines these qualities is available, it must be accepted that if the first requirement is fulfilled the problem of condensation must be reduced by adequate ventilation.

Plain brick walls are not satisfactory, since bricks are absorbent and do not provide a really smooth surface even when the mortar joints are finished flush with the face of the wall.

Plastered walls, especially if finished with a final coat of hard plaster covered with a high-gloss paint, will overcome the irregularity of the structural material of the wall and provide a jointless and reasonably non-porous surface. Matt finishes are somewhat less liable to cause condensation. Soft plaster and lath and stud partitions should not be used; this type of construction is liable to harbour rats and mice, which may break into the cavity by gnawing through the skirting-board. Proprietary anti-condensation plasters are obtainable; their surfaces have an open texture which rapidly assumes air temperature and accordingly prevents condensation, if a reasonable air humidity is maintained. Certain paints are effective too, up to a point, and also linings of expanded polystyrene, although the latter is very soft and easily broken down on walls.

Match-boards are most unsuitable for wall surfaces. They may shrink or swell, and their joints collect dirt. They are easily penetrated by rodents, and those with hollow backs provide an excellent harbour for pests. Fibre-board sheets have considerable insulating value and are not conducive to condensation unless hard faced, but they are not pest-proof and will not withstand frequent washing. The basic materials are wood pulp or root or cane fibre, sawmill waste, straw, waste paper, bark and similar vegetable fibres. Although sheets of these materials may be used in large sizes, joints are unavoidable when wall surfaces are covered. The use of cover slips or battens over the joints is undesirable since they form a minor dirt pocket. It is better for the joints to be covered with a strip of hessian 'scrim', and the whole surface 'floated' with plaster or covered with plastic paint. All these materials are absorbent and not readily cleaned. They soak up grease, dirt and moisture and they are impervious and should not be used where open food is prepared, stored or sold.

Materials with a vitreous surface include glazed tiles, glass tiles, glass bricks and various proprietary opaque glass or mirror panels. Of these, glazed tiles are preferable; although made in a small unit size, the joints are fine, smooth and flush, whereas other types must be screwed into place and it may be necessary to use cover slips at the joints.

Other hard-surface panels are made of asbestos-cement sheets or plastic sheets. With all hard panels a wall surface of excellent hygienic quality is obtainable, but raised covers for joints and projections due to fixing methods should be avoided.

Ceilings

As a general rule it is desirable for roofs or floors over food-preparation rooms to be underdrawn or ceiled. It is probable that the traditional and most common material, plaster, is suitable in most situations, although other materials have advantages in certain circumstances. Ceilings, as distinct from the undersides of roofs or upper floors, serve four purposes: they provide a smooth non-dust-collecting internal surface to the room, prevent dust filtering down into the room through the upper floor or roof, improve the degree of insulation of the roof, and provide a level undersurface with no pockets in which hot humid air can collect and stagnate.

Fibre-boards provide better insulation than plaster; they are self-supporting and more easily fixed in some conditions, for example, by patent clips to the underside of light corrugated sheet roofs with steel frames. Patent anti-condensation plasters which incorporate porous but non-permeable materials reduce the rate of thermal transmission and have relatively warm surfaces. Tiles or slabs of expanded polystyrene (foamed plastic) can be readily fixed to the underside of ceilings; they reduce condensation substantially. The use of polystyrene tiles, under certain conditions, presents a fire hazard; they should not be painted with gloss paint.

Decorative finishes for walls and ceilings

The hot and humid atmosphere in kitchens frequently plays havoc with wall and ceiling paints and distempers, and causes surfaces to blister, peel and flake. Wherever walls, not constructed of impervious material, may be splashed with greasy water, a non-absorbent washable coat of paint or good oilbound distemper is essential; above this line an easily renewed and light medium, such as whitening or colour-wash, should be maintained. 1·8 metres (6 feet) above floor level is suggested as a suitable height for a washable dado. To reduce condensation, there should be adequate ventilation, natural or artificial, particularly over cookers, boilers, sinks and similar installations.

Granulated cork has long been painted on the walls and ceilings of crews' quarters in ships to minimize condensation, and proprietary paints incorporating powdered cork are being used successfully in kitchens for this same purpose.

Lighting

In general, there is no obligatory standard of lighting for kitchens in the UK; from observations in many establishments it may be questioned whether an enforceable standard is not necessary, as a particularly good system of lighting is essential. The code of the United States prescribes a minimum illumination equal to 20 foot-candles on working surfaces; the Regulations of the Department of Education and Science relating to kitchens attached to schools in England and Wales impose a similar requirement and a daylight factor of 2. This amount of light should not be difficult to attain by natural light on medium days, providing the windows are not overshadowed by nearby buildings, and from modern artificial sources.

Although there are other illuminants which have their uses in very remote places or temporary situations, electric current is now generally available. Both tungsten filament lamps and strip (fluorescent) lighting are in common use. Although more expensive to install, the strip lighting is more economical in current consumption. A tungsten lamp is cheaper to replace and it gives best light when used with a reflector fitting such as the British Standard Specification (BSS) 232-1926 or the Department of the Environment (formerly Ministry of Works) A36. Light bulbs should have some form of shade or cover, in order to prevent the scatter or splinters of glass in the event of bulbs fragmenting. Shades should be chosen carefully so that there is minimal loss of light.

Lighting points should be directly above sinks and food-preparation benches. Preferably, they should be set back 456 mm

(18 inches) from the front of the sink towards the wall, so that the person who is washing up casts no shadow on the contents of the sink.

It is not only working surfaces which need adequate lighting; no part of the premises should be so dark that it is difficult to see whether utensils are clean or not. If the food room is reasonably spacious for the work performed, convenient in shape and lay-out, and decorated in light colours, then a system of lighting which is satisfactory for working surfaces should meet the needs of other parts of the room by diffusion. Direct sunlight is likely to be tiresome to the eyes of the workers, and in food-preparation rooms it is also a source of undesirable warmth to perishable foods. For these reasons, windows on a north wall are preferable; otherwise, precautions, such as the use of obscured glass or window blinds, should be taken to obtain indirect lighting.

Ventilation

For ordinary purposes, the natural ventilation of buildings is sufficient except in rooms which are over-populated. The vaporous

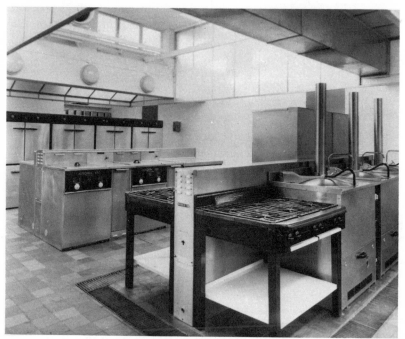

Fig. 41. Efficient and hygienic grouping of equipment

products of cooking, however, can rarely be effectively removed from a kitchen except by means of mechanical extraction.

The British Standards Institution recommends (1950) that provision should be made for up to 20 air changes per hour in large kitchens, and it is obvious that natural ventilation could not secure this rate of air change. It is suggested that such frequent change of the air in a kitchen is neither necessary nor desirable, nor the most satisfactory method of controlling humidity and cooking

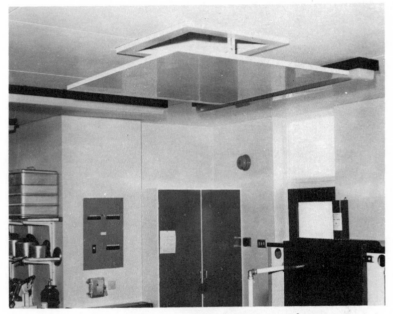

Fig. 42.   Baffle board centred over extract duct

odours. Far greater efficiency is obtained by strictly localized systems of extraction, analogous to the methods employed to remove dust from grinding and polishing machines.

The grouping of cooking appliances in islands is a convenient method of concentrating this equipment to enable the cooking odours and steam to be removed before they are diffused throughout the kitchen. The equipment shown in Fig. 41 is blocked or boned together like unit furniture with all services concealed in a central chamber; it is a most successful and hygienic lay-out.

Although the traditional canopy and extraction fans are still highly efficient methods of extraction, they do visually interrupt the kitchen space and cause cleaning problems. Simple baffle boards placed below extraction fans are now being used with evident success. The boards, usually made from block-boards, plastic-laminate covered, are about 1 metre (1 yard) square and suspended below the ceiling on adjustable straps. The distance

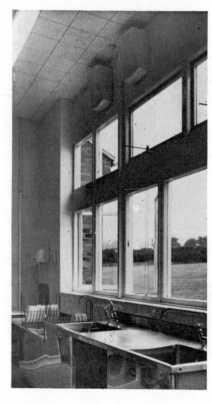

Fig. 43.

Vent-Axia
extraction fans

between the baffle board and the ceiling can easily be adjusted until the required extract velocity is achieved. The whole baffle board can easily be removed, cleaned and replaced within minutes (Fig. 42). Ducting is reduced to a minimum, especially if the extraction fan is roof mounted.

As a supplement to open windows or permanently open grills, small electric extraction fans are suitable for small kitchens (Fig. 43); they should be at a distance from an air inlet to prevent air from short-circuiting them. Installations of this type can be used over the wash-up sinks which contribute to humidity in kitchens.

Café bars usually have a tea boiler on the counter, and the flue discharges into the air of the room. There is often a hood or dome suspended above this, but without a duct or trunk leading to the open air. As a means of preventing general condensation in the room, it is useless; but it breaks up and diffuses concentrations of heat and water vapour, which would otherwise impinge upon a small area of ceiling immediately above the flue, thus causing rapid deterioration of decorations.

Sanitary convenience and washing facilities

In common with other premises where persons are employed, buildings where food is handled must be provided with sufficient water-closets, urinals, and wash-hand-basins for the use of the staff, and in all but the smallest restaurants it may be a requirement (see Public Health Act, 1936, section 89) to provide sanitary accommodation for members of the public using the building. As to the number of sanitary conveniences considered necessary, the Sanitary Convenience Regulations, 1964, set out in considerable detail the number of water-closets and urinals to be provided in relation to the number of employees. In general, the provision of a sanitary convenience for every multiple of 15 males or females will meet the requirements, but in special cases reference should be made to the Schedule in the Regulations.

Where more than 10 females are employed, suitable provision must also be made for the disposal of sanitary dressings. If there is a solid fuel boiler in constant use on the premises, sanitary dressings can be burnt, and pedal-operated binettes may be used in the toilets. Gas-fired or electric sanitary incinerators may be installed, although the flues of these appliances sometimes cause trouble. As an alternative, chemical incinerators are now in use; they require attention from time to time.

Premises which are licensed by county councils as places of entertainment are required to provide sanitary conveniences for the public. In the former county of Middlesex, for example, for every 1,000 of the total number of persons to be accommodated, there must be 2 WCs and 5 urinals for men, and 4 WCs for women. A similar standard could be applied to catering establishments seating, say, 200 persons or more.

The standard washdown pedestal pan is adequate for installation

in food premises but where low-level flushing suites are used, a
siphonic pan is recommended for more positive clearance. By a
simple adaptation, low-level cisterns may be flushed by a foot-
pedal—a commendable and hygienic arrangement (Fig. 44).

The siting of sanitary conveniences in relation to work-rooms,
habitable rooms and rooms in which food is prepared has long been
the subject of statutory control; conveniences must not be placed in
food rooms or, indeed, in direct communication with them. Any
water-closet or urinal used in connection with a food room must,

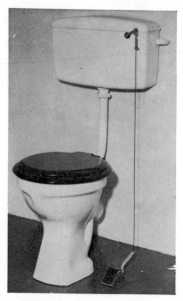 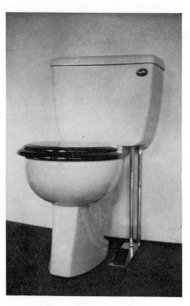

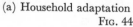

(a) Household adaptation   (b) Permanent installation
FIG. 44.   Foot-operated flush

therefore, be entered either from the open air or through some
intervening and separately ventilated lobby. This arrangement is
enforced nowadays and the lobby is frequently and sensibly
utilized by fitting one or more hand-wash-basins. Because it is
important for a food handler to wash after visiting the toilet, it is
imperative that a wash-basin should be near the conveniences.
A worker's hands may also become dirty, and indeed contaminated, from raw foods and other materials during the course of
the day, so that additional wash-basins provided solely for this
purpose should be placed conveniently in the food room (Fig. 45).

When food handlers are engaged in work on more than one floor of a multi-storied building, conveniences and adjacent wash-hand-basins are desirable on each storey; they should, at least, be situated so that each serves not more than two floors. Water-closet apartments must be adequately lighted and ventilated either by natural or artificial means.

Appliances for hand washing may comprise fixed wash-basins, troughs, or washing fountains (circular bowls at least 0·9 metre (3 feet) in diameter). With troughs, a length of 0·6 metre (2 feet) is regarded as equivalent to a wash-basin; with fountains, 0·6 metre

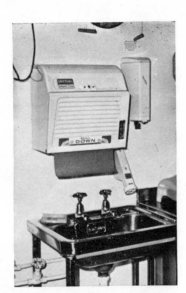

FIG. 45.   Hand-wash-basin, plus paper towels, in a kitchen

(2 feet) of circumference is allowed. Foot-operated water control (Fig. 46) is recommended for food factories.

The Washing Facilities Regulations, 1964, require basins or their equivalent in troughs or fountains to be provided on the same scale as sanitary conveniences.

Where bakers and pastry-cooks are employed in kitchens, the Welfare Order of 1927, applicable to Bakehouses and Biscuit Factories, are of interest; they prescribe 1 wash-hand-basin of a depth not less than 178 mm and a length not less than 500 mm (7 and 20 inches) for every 10 employees. It should be noted that these orders are concerned primarily with safeguarding the health of the employees (against dermatitis in this case) rather than the transmission of disease to the public; hence the specified dimensions of the basins, which are intended to permit cleansing not only of the hands but also of the forearms.

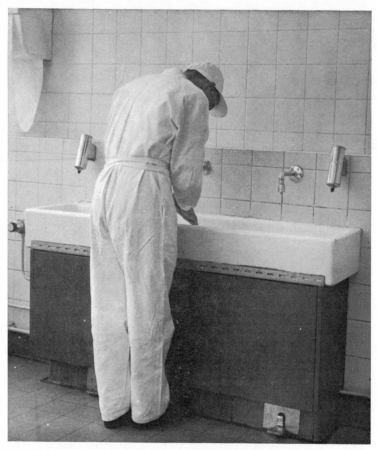

FIG. 46.   Foot-operated water control and sprinkler

For hand washing there must be supplies of running hot and cold water, or water blended to a suitable temperature. In premises where there is a central boiler-fed hot-water system the distribution of hot water to wash-hand-basins is not difficult. When a piped supply of hot water is not available there are several excellent alternatives, such as thermal storage units and instantaneous water heaters using electricity or gas as a source of heat.

Spray taps which discharge water at a temperature of 48·9 °C (about 120 °F) are economical in the volume of water delivered and consequently in the amount of fuel required for heating. Lever-arm taps, as installed in hospitals, which can be operated by the elbow or forearm, greatly reduce chances of cross-contamination; alternatively, pedal-operated taps or sprinkers should be used (Fig. 46).

Washing facilities do not, of course, finish at the provision of water and basins; soap, in tablet form, or perhaps better still as powder or liquid from a fitted dispenser, is necessary; also nail brushes and some means to dry the hands. The most hygienic methods are provided by paper towels which can be destroyed after use, the continuous roller towel when each portion is used once only, and the many types of hot-air hand driers.

Drainage

The design and general construction of drainage systems are regulated for all kinds of building. Of special though not exclusive application to food-preparation rooms is the prohibition of discharging obstructive matter into drains (Public Health Act, 1936, section 27). Certain waste products of food preparation are likely to lead to choked drains. For example, the fat and grease from washing-up water are discharged hot and molten; they rapidly cool during their passage through the drain and solidify there unless intercepted. Grease traps are tanks which hold a volume of cold water, sufficient in quantity to cool any inflow of dish water to below the melting point of its grease content. Inlets and outlets are submerged so that the solidified fat forms a floating curd which must be skimmed off as the need arises. Nevertheless, grease traps are not always satisfactory; if correct procedures and materials are used the problem of grease should rarely arise.

The use of fat-solvent detergents changes the nature of the retained fat from a fairly hard set and brittle skin to a sticky crumb, which does not readily separate from the water and is thus less easily removed; it may be necessary to pump it out and carry it away for disposal by contractors. Furthermore, it appears to be no longer acceptable for any manufacturing process.

It is claimed that the inoculation of sink waste in a specially constructed tank with a preparation of bacterial enzymes liquefies the grease, so that the waste can be safely discharged into the drainage system.

The accepted way to drain kitchens is to sink glazed stoneware channels into the floor in suitable positions, so that waste water can be carried away to a gully situated outside the building. Where the channels cross the open floor a cover-grid should be provided, preferably of galvanized or zinc-sprayed cast iron, to avoid accidents. The grid must be in short lengths and easily removed to allow regular and frequent cleansing of the channel. Sinks and wash-hand-basins should discharge properly into or over gullies. Fresh air inlets and ventilation pipes connected to drainage systems are not allowed in food rooms; furthermore, every inlet into such a system must be trapped.

Refuse storage

Unlike the scrap from many industrial and commercial processes, kitchen waste demands particular care and attention while awaiting final disposal, owing to its putrescible nature and the special needs of kitchen premises.

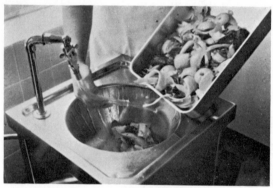

FIG. 47.   Waste disposal unit

Undoubtedly, the principle of immediate disposal of kitchen waste by disintegration and flushing to the drainage system, or by direct incineration, is attractive hygienically. Unfortunately, the costs of installation and running equipment for this purpose may be considered rather high for the smaller catering business.

Waste disposal units which discharge into the drainage system may be fixed under metal sinks or stand in a frame with their own receiving hoppers. An electrically driven macerating unit breaks down waste food to a fine mash which is washed away through a trapped waste pipe. In one type the machine is automatically switched on only when water is flowing through the grinding chamber (Fig. 47). Units designed for the domestic market have motors of 1/3 h.p. but generally a heavier duty motor should be used in commercial premises.

Some waste materials cause breakdowns in the units; string and cloth, for example, become entangled in the grinder and cans dent or fold and jam the machine; glass and soft bones, however, can be reduced to fine particles.

Incineration must not be accompanied by the emission of smoke or odour and accordingly must take place under conditions of total combustion. For this purpose, incinerators are specially designed

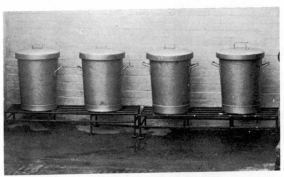

FIG. 48.   Dustbins on stands

with additional heat supplied by an auxiliary fuel such as gas or oil, applied not only in the combustion chamber, but also as an 'after-burner' in the flue gas stream.

The use of chutes directly to the incinerator or to the place of storage is undesirable for unwrapped wet refuse.

Used cans with food particles still adhering to the inside are often attractive to flies, and their bulk, pending removal, presents a storage problem. However, these difficulties can be lessened. Small cans approximately 0·45 kg (1 lb) in size may be flattened by a specially designed press, but larger cans need balers which would not usually be available in any but the largest establishments. The modern packaging materials such as foil and polystyrene are bulky; they are difficult to store prior to collection and their ultimate disposal is not easy.

Whatever method of disposal is chosen the storage of certain waste or refuse which cannot be dealt with on the premises is necessary.

There are many advantages in the system of storage in paper sacks which are now being marketed by many companies. Several forms of stand are available for holding the sack, and hinged lids are provided to protect the open sack fitted in the holder (Fig. 49). Whilst they are fairly waterproof, the sacks should not be used for wet unwrapped waste; when they are outside it is preferable but not essential to have overhead covers. Obviously, they are not suitable for hot ashes. The filled sacks are light and clean to handle, they have a good means of closure and, from the collector's point of view, they do not need a special vehicle for transportation. Some local

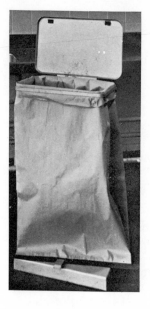

Fig. 49.   Paper sack and holder

councils provide householders with plastic sacks for refuse and schools sometimes buy their own supplies.

Dustbins must be made of stout impervious material and 22 gauge galvanized iron is recommended. They should be cylindrical with a slight taper to a narrower bottom to ease the work of disposal and to avoid dents. The thickness of the metal rather than the corrugations supplies the strength. The bin should not exceed 0·05 cubic metre (2 cubic feet) in capacity and it should be provided with suitable handles. The close-fitting lid must have a deep lip, at least 50 mm (2 inches) as a precaution against disturbance by wind or marauding cats and dogs; lids of hard rubber substantially reduce noise when the bins are being used. There is a British Standard Specification for the construction of dustbins.

For an economic and effective life, the bin must be used carefully. It should not be filled to overflowing, so that the lid balances on a pile of exposed refuse, and after it has been emptied the bin should be scrubbed or hosed inside and out and left to drain dry. As far as possible wet refuse should be wrapped in newspaper or other waste paper; this enables the bin to be emptied cleanly without rough handling.

The amount of storage space required for refuse depends partly on the frequency of collection. The usual interval between collections is 7 days. It may be daily in some areas, but during the fly season it should not be longer than 3 days, particularly for food waste. It is not always practicable to place the dustbins on a site which is convenient for both the refuse collector and the occupier of the premises. Where the dustbins are some distance from the food room and scraps are kept in the room, a suitable covered vessel should be used and emptied into the bins at least at the close of each day; plastic binettes with pedal-operated lids, or paper sacks are suitable for this purpose.

Yards belonging to food premises should be properly paved and drained, and this is particularly necessary for the ground which provides the site for the refuse bin. A stand for the bins constructed of iron rods or angle iron to allow a clearance under the bins of about 229 mm (9 inches) is an advantage (Fig. 48). This extra height is helpful when the bins have to be lifted for emptying, but the main purpose of the arrangement is to allow the yard pavement to be properly hosed down and swept.

Equipment

Just as the surface of the walls and floors must be of a texture which is easily cleaned, so all surfaces with which food comes in contact must allow for thorough cleaning almost to a state of sterility. The ease with which any item of food equipment can be cleaned depends upon the extent to which its material and design provide lodgement for food scraps in parts which are difficult to reach. The basic material for food equipment must be non-absorbent and not subject to injury by cleaning or by any of the bactericidal agents which are available. Separate cutting blocks and 'boards' should be used for different foods, particularly for raw and cooked foods, to lower the risk of cross-contamination.

Wooden tops to work benches, wooden draining boards and teak sinks were for many years popular in the catering trade. They are difficult to clean and likely to retain bacteria in cracks and corners. Experiments have shown that large numbers of intestinal bacteria may be cultivated from teak sinks even after thorough washing and scrubbing with a strong soda solution. Wooden equipment is therefore unsuitable for food work. It can be satisfactorily replaced by alternative materials such as linoleum bonded on wood, plastic or metal table tops, and 'jointless' metal combined sinks and draining boards or glazed-ware sinks, but the overhanging lip of a draining board should be avoided.

The Food Hygiene (General) Regulations 1970 require such surfaces to be made of materials unable to absorb matter. There are now alternative materials to wood for the butcher's block. Where wooden blocks are used, they are usually cleansed by scraping followed by scrubbing with detergent; a final wipe with a cloth wrung out in hypochlorite solution is recommended. In former days, and perhaps in some instances now, water was not applied to blocks but the surface was scraped and salted periodically. The better blocks are made of hard woods such as maple or hornbeam, so that washing and scrubbing ought not to affect them unduly. Cutting boards should be constructed from one piece of wood without joints; after use they should be washed and scrubbed thoroughly with detergent and hypochlorite.

Alternative materials for cutting surfaces are now available. Compressed rubber slabs and also boards covered with a sheet of plastic are often used. They are more easily cleaned and therefore more hygienic, but the plastic may be dangerous for large-scale work because the surface becomes slippery for meat and knives.

Cooking vessels and other utensils may be made of a wide range of material, including various metals and vitreous substances. There have been no reports of illness following the consumption of foodstuffs prepared in contact with the more common metals such as aluminium and its alloys, iron, tin or stainless steel. Zinc poisoning, however, has been reported in two incidents where apple rings were prepared in a galvanized iron container, and outbreaks of chemical poisoning from lemonade prepared in chipped enamel containers provide examples of antimony poisoning. Copper from tea urns and from tin-coated steamers from which the tin layer has been worn has been reported as a cause of chemical food poisoning.

Equipment should be placed so that it can be easily cleaned from all sides and should be at least 300 mm (12 inches) away from walls. If it is in a central position, enough room should be left to allow entrance to the backs of adjacent ranges and similar equipment. There should be provision for in-plant cleaning for parts of equipment that are fixed and yet subject to food debris. Small pieces of equipment such as mixing machines can be mobile on small trolleys (Fig. 50).

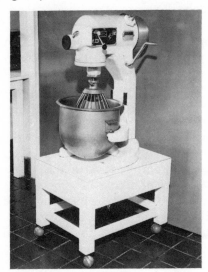

FIG. 50. Food mixer mounted on mobile table

Design and installation

It is not always possible to provide an unbroken smooth surface for parts of equipment or appliances with which food comes into contact, however obviously desirable this may be, but dirt traps such as lips or ledges, projections, crevices and acute internal angles should be reduced to an unavoidable minimum.

Equipment with moving parts, for example mixers, mincers and slicers, frequently present difficulties in the way of thorough cleaning, and machines of these and similar kinds should be selected on the basis of ease of dismantling and reassembly.

General dirt is liable to accumulate in the framework and outer casings of appliances, which again should be as smooth as practicable, and spaces in the supporting structure should either be totally enclosed and sealed or fully open to allow good access for cleaning. For example, legs to standing equipment are better when formed of sealed tubes rather than of angle or channel section and there should be an open space, some 300 mm (12 inches) high, under the appliance for ease of cleaning; but where the working height and the depth of the fixture do not allow for an adequate open space beneath, it should be mounted or sealed to a solid base, such as a concrete plinth 100 to 150 mm (4 to 6 inches) high topped with quarry tiles and with a coved tile skirting.

To enable proper cleaning of floors and walls, bulky equipment which is not easily moveable should stand 300 mm (12 inches) from any wall, and when appliances are grouped back-to-back in islands, similar provision should be made between each item. Service pipes should be encased to prevent the accumulation of dirt and insects, or chased into the walls, or covered or taken out in service ducts.

Hot water supply

The hot water requirements of food-preparation rooms vary both in quantity and temperature, and may have to be met in different ways even within the same premises. It may be said that the basic needs are small quantities of boiling water for tea-making, medium amounts of warm water 48·9 °C (about 120 °F) for hand washing, large quantities of hot water 60 to 65·6 °C (140 to 150 °F) for utensil washing and provision for a disinfecting rinse 82·2 °C (180 °F).

The tea boiler is almost invariably an independent gas-burning instantaneous heater, of which there are several types made by various manufacturers.

Hot water installations do not usually provide a supply of water at sterilizing temperatures unless specifically designed for the purpose, and not all appliances on the market are capable of doing so. For this reason water for hand washing and for dishes is often supplied independently, either from storage at 65·6 °C (150 °F) after heating by independent solid fuel, oil, gas or electrically heated boiler, by indirect heating from a steam or hot-water central-heating system, or by delivery from an instantaneous gas water heater. When such a supply, piped or otherwise, is provided, it is a relatively simple matter to raise the temperature of the water in the sink used for the disinfecting rinse by means of a thermostatically controlled gas burner or electrical unit or by steam. This reduces loss of heat from the rinse water while work is in progress. Another system which has been used successfully to overcome this difficulty is the provision of water, heated to 82·2 °C (180 °F) by an independent boiler, directly to the disinfecting sink from which there may be a constant overflow to the washing sink as the water cools.

For hand-washing supplies, where a piped supply is not practicable from the main hot-water system, small gas geysers or electric thermal storage appliances are invaluable, but they must not be expected to supply water at high temperatures for washing-up.

15

Control of Infestation

(*The late L. KLUTH*)

It is probable that estimates of the material damage caused by rats and mice are often overstated, and the implication of these rodents in the spread of infection in Britain is probably not considerable, although not insignificant, at the present time. Nevertheless, the presence of such animals in and around food stores is repugnant, apart from being a source of material loss and a potential danger to health.

Local authorities invariably maintain a staff of pest operators trained in methods of rodent destruction, and the occupier of infested premises can call for practical assistance. It should be pointed out that the onus for keeping premises free from infestation rests upon the occupier, and councils are entitled to charge for such services. Where there is serious damage to food caused by any infestation the occupier is under an obligation to report it to the authorities (Prevention of Damage by Pests Act, 1949, section 13).

Block control of rats and mice

The Black death (fourteenth century) was bubonic plague caused by *Pasteurella pestis* which was spread from rat to rat and from rat to man by fleas carrying the organisms; 25 million people died. Certain countries still suffer this disease. The rat is clever, breeds prolifically, gnaws voraciously and may carry agents of other diseases such as leptospirosis and viral and food-borne infections.

An infestation is not always confined to one part of a building which may be occupied by different families or firms, nor to a single building; the rat or mouse colony may spread through several adjoining premises. In this case a tenant might kill off the rodents on his own premises, only to find them replaced in a very short time by an overflow from his neighbour's property. Concerted action over the whole infested territory or block is necessary before all the rats and mice can be destroyed. Usually this is carried out most conveniently by the local authority and it is known as block control (Fig. 51).

216

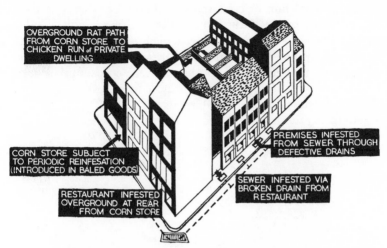

FIG. 51. Block control: an example of related infestation in separate buildings which require simultaneous treatment

Vertical block control

An infestation may extend below ground to drains and sewers, so that vertical block control schemes must include treatment for the destruction of rats in underground pipes as well as in the buildings above.

Rat-proofing

Some comment has already been made (p. 195–198) on structural materials and their properties of resistance to penetration by rodents. Naturally, stony and metallic materials have basic advantages over those of a fibrous nature. Impenetrable materials, however, are of little value if the building is constructed so that apertures or cavities are left for rodents to use as a means of entry or passage or as a place to nest in. Furthermore, thoughtless methods of food storage, careless stacking and general untidiness may allow a considerable infestation to become established in an otherwise sealed building; a rat or mouse family may be introduced through the store entrance, for example, in straw packing materials.

The major requirements for survival and family life in the rodent world are food, water and housing, and to deny any or all of these is a means of discouraging infestation. Therefore, material which is likely to be suitable for rat food, e.g. cereals, starchy vegetables and fatty compounds, including even tallow and soap, should be kept in rat-proof metal bins or containers, and refuse of the same type in properly covered metal dustbins, whilst awaiting removal. As far as possible access to water should be denied by attending to dripping taps and keeping grids on gully traps, for example. Articles temporarily unused should not be allowed to accumulate in odd corners nor remain undisturbed for more than a week or two, thus providing refuge for rats; anything which may afford cover to rats should be eliminated from the building and attached yards.

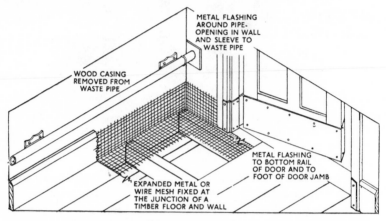

Fig. 52.   Rat-proofing: methods of protecting some vulnerable points

Where there are quantitities of cartons or boxed goods they should be neatly stacked close together, either immediately against a wall or at least 0·6 metre (2 feet) from it, as rats hesitate to cross open spaces.

Drains often provide an entrance to a building and should be maintained in good repair with all inlets, manholes and rodding eyes properly sealed or covered. There are other vulnerable points such as broken air-gratings in walls, openings for pipe-work sometimes below ground, ill-fitting doors, worn thresholds, the gnawed bottoms and jambs of doors and corrugation in the wall or roof. Structural harbours may occur below hollow floors, in hollow walls and partitions, in pipe ducts and casings and less commonly in roof spaces.

Figure 52 illustrates remedies for some of the common defects mentioned above. It shows some of the means by which the passage of rats from one part of a building to another (for example, from a subfloor space and the room above) may be prevented. It will be seen that to proof a building against rats, openings must be sealed by cement mortar, sheet metal or mesh. Similar materials should reinforce vulnerable points such as door edges and junction points of walls and floors.

Rat destruction

Rats are creatures of habit and suspicious by nature; they avoid new objects.

Rats may be trapped, but poisoning, when practised methodically, is generally more wholesale in effect.

A good measure of success has been achieved for some years by the use in suitable bait (e.g. oatmeal) of a material known as 'Warfarin' which, after several doses, prevents the coagulation of blood and produces spontaneous haemorrhage. During the feeding period of 3 to 8 days before death, the rat appears to experience no pain or significant loss of appetite and no 'bait-shyness' develops. As the poisoned bait is acceptable immediately, no pre-baiting is carried out, but it must be replenished or renewed for a period up to 10 days. The proportion of Warfarin used in the bait is small, giving a final concentration of toxicant of 0·025 per cent, so that there is a large margin of safety in case of accidental ingestion by man or domestic animals. Also, as the poison is effective only after repeated doses the danger to creatures other than rodents is remote. It is considered advisable however, to lay the baits in containers or in positions readily accessible to rodents only; thus the bait, approximately 85 g (3 oz) should be laid in established and currently used rat runs.

Populations of rats in various parts of the UK have become resistant to Warfarin; resistance is reported in Denmark also. Where such a position arises, the selective destruction of non-resistant strains by the continued use of an anticoagulant reduces the natural competition amongst the rats in a neighbourhood, and can lead to a less restricted reproduction and overflow of resistant rat colonies into wider areas.

As an alternative, zinc phosphide may be used. This poison is subject to the Poisons Rules for purchase and use, and should only be handled by a trained operator; care must be taken to ensure that food or water for human consumption does not become contaminated. These rules apply also to arsenious oxide, which should not be placed in dwelling houses or where food is handled. The use of these poisons is regrettable as they cannot be considered humane. The vasoconstrictor Norbormide is relatively painless. It is a selective rat toxicant, expensive but effective; it is not toxic to mice. Poisonous dusts such as lindane may be used; the rat picks up the dust on its feet and fur and the poison is ingested by the action of grooming, since the rat is clean in its personal habits.

Fluoroacetamide is a rodenticide; it is subject to the Poisons Rules and may be used only by fully trained operators, in ships or sewers; it should never be used in agriculture, horticulture, the home or any place where food is handled. Many of these poisons are not recommended, except in emergencies, for humane reasons.

Mice

The mouse appears to be less a creature of habit than the rat, less suspicious of unfamiliar objects and less consistent in travel routes and established feeding points. Thus the individual trap may be quite useful, whilst wholesale extermination by poisoning may be less effective than for rats. Mice, or as they are sometimes called 'supermice', appear to be on the increase, due to resistance to poisons such as Warfarin.

Of all traps, the spring break-back type is most used although it suffers from the disadvantage that once sprung it is of no further use until reset. A substantial number of traps set in a mouse-infested area over a period of several nights usually has a good effect. A treadle or plate is better for holding bait than a prong because cereal bait such as oatmeal, flour or breadcrumbs may be used and, contrary to popular belief, they are more attractive to mice than the traditional cheese. It is desirable to place the bait so that the striker will hit the animal's head. If the bait is scattered, the frequency of maiming is increased.

Baits containing 0·25 per cent of Warfarin and in quantities of 28 g (1 oz) are also used with reasonable success against mice, although resistance is developing. A new poison, Alphachloralose, is now in use; it kills quickly and humanely. The metabolic rate is reduced and the mice die from heat loss. Alphachloralose is used indoors only where temperatures are low (less than 18 °C; 65 °F); at higher temperatures mice recover from the stupefying condition. A contact dust based on lindane is also used for mice.

The Animals (Cruel Poisons) Act, 1962

Red squill, phosphorus and strychnine have been prohibited by a regulation under the above-mentioned Act, and certain other poisons may eventually be prohibited in the same way. Thallium compounds are dangerous to human life besides being very inhumane; permits for their use must be obtained from the medical officer of health.

Flies

House-flies, bluebottles and greenbottles, once so prevalent and potentially dangerous, are nowadays less significant as a result of two major changes in our way of life over the past half century. These changes are, firstly, the disappearance of horse-drawn traffic, and the consequent diminution in the amount of horse manure, which is the fly's first choice of breeding ground; secondly, the water-carriage system of drainage in use throughout urban areas, which greatly reduces the risk of access by flies to infectious material.

In spite of these improvements there are often far too many flies about in their season, and any uncovered and undisturbed vegetable refuse, fish and meat offal can serve as breeding grounds. The chance that a fly may spread communicable diseases by infecting food is a possibility and there are circumstances where flies may gain access to infected material. For example, in earth closets or pail closets where they are still used, in crêches and day nurseries where very young children are still at the 'pot' stage, at slaughterhouses and knackers' yards, and in places where there are stools of rats, mice, cats, dogs and other animals which may excrete food-poisoning organisms. Food should be protected from contamination by flies.

Whilst the danger of fly-borne contamination of food must not be over-emphasized, and certainly not to the extent of diverting the public mind from the really vital safeguards of personal cleanliness, animal husbandry and refrigeration, it would not be safe to ignore completely the possibility and all steps should be taken to deny flies access to food intended for human consumption.

Four methods of approach may be suggested, but since none of these is likely to be effective independently, a combination of all four should be practised. Control may be exercised (a) by the elimination of breeding places, (b) by measures to destroy the fly at some period of its life cycle, (c) by protecting foodstuffs, or better still by making food premises fly-proof as far as practicable, and (d) by obtaining practical advice from the public health inspector.

The elimination of breeding places is the responsibility of the food trader, but others have a duty in the matter too. Refuse is universal and the public should be aware of the sources of material used by flies for breeding, so that they too may play a part in its control. Likewise the local authorities should be vigilant in detecting and dealing with accumulations of offensive material. With modern methods of on-site disposal, refuse collection and the availability of suitable refuse containers, there is no reason why waste which is attractive to flies should be left putrefying and uncovered anywhere.

Measures against flies, as with all pests, depend primarily on a knowledge of the life-cycle and habits of the insects. In common with many other species, the house-fly passes through four stages, the time spent in each depending upon weather conditions, especially temperature. The stages are: (1) the egg, which is laid by the female in some material which provides food for (2) the larva or maggot which hatches from the egg after 8 hours to 3 days. The larva burrows into its food supply, eating vigorously until fully grown, which takes from 42 hours to as much as 6 to 8 weeks, when it seeks a dry and cool spot in which to pupate. The pupa (3) or chrysalis remains motionless in its cocoon for a period of 3 days to 4 weeks when (4) the adult fly emerges.

The two most vulnerable states are those of the larva and the adult, when the creature is mobile. Migrating maggots may be destroyed by boiling water or contact insecticides, and where manure bins are used there should be a larva-trap either beneath or around them. Although there are many forms of fly-trap and many poisons, the most effective way to destroy flies is by insecticidal sprays containing natural or synthetic pyrethrins, BHC, fenitrothion or dichlorvos. Liberated as a fine mist, the spray of pyrethrins activated with piperonyl butoxide immediately kills flies on the wing. The other compounds in higher concentrations and sprayed on walls, ceilings and hanging fixtures have a residual action, killing flies which come in contact with the surfaces over a period of weeks. Deposits of insecticides on food or on equipment in direct contact with food must be avoided because of possible toxic effects. Aerosol devices which release pyrethrins at regular intervals and resin strips impregnated with dichlorvos can be used to control flying insects.

There is a danger from 'knock-down' insecticides; insects affected in flight may drop into adjacent food mixes and escape detection. A type of electrical device uses ultra-violet fluorescent tubes as a lure to attract insects on to an electrified grid; the insects are immediately killed and fall into a collecting tray.

Thorough cleanliness and an absence of uncovered food scraps both inside and outside the kitchen will make the premises less attractive to flies. Whilst it is not always easy to fly-proof premises, at least all external doors should be self-closing and windows

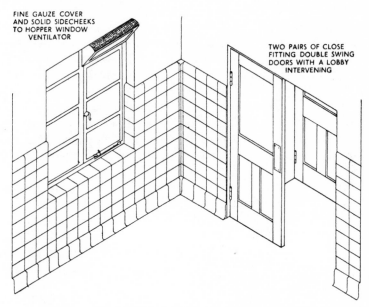

FINE GAUZE COVER
AND SOLID SIDECHEEKS
TO HOPPER WINDOW
VENTILATOR

TWO PAIRS OF CLOSE
FITTING DOUBLE SWING
DOORS WITH A LOBBY
INTERVENING

FIG. 53.   Fly-proofing: protecting common places of entry

and ventilators covered with fine gauze (Fig. 53). It is said that a net, which moves in the wind, may be hung loosely over doorways to exclude flies for even though the mesh be quite large flies fear entanglement; hanging plastic strips are used widely on the Continent for the same purpose. In buildings which are not fully proofed against flies—and many are not—larders should be safeguarded and displayed foods covered; crockery and cutlery should be protected after cleaning.

Cockroaches

Cockroaches most commonly found in this country are the Oriental cockroach or black beetle and the German cockroach or steam-fly, which is light yellow-brown in colour. The two species are not often present in one building at the same time. They are both nocturnal in habit, occupy crevices in walls and floors, especially in warm places, and they are catholic in their choice of foodstuffs, with a notable taste for beer. Hitherto they have rarely been implicated in outbreaks of disease; nevertheless, salmonella organisms were isolated from cockroaches infesting a children's ward in a hospital where there had been an extensive outbreak of gastroenteritis. The creatures are known to carry other organisms, dysentery and tubercle bacilli and the cholera vibrio.

Before commencing an insecticidal treatment it is important to determine the extent of the infestation by means of a thorough inspection carried out after dark when the premises are quiet. Cockroaches are readily repelled by some insecticides and for this reason treatment should start beyond the infested area so that insects attempting to disperse cannot avoid contact with the insecticide.

Cockroaches are susceptible to most classes of insecticide, including organochlorines (BHC, dieldrin, chlordane and chlordecone), organophosphates (fenitrothion, diazinon, iodofenphos), carbamates (propoxur, bendicarb, dioxacarb), and pyrethroids (pyrethrins, resmethrin). These insecticides are formulated and can be applied in various ways to make optimal use of their properties. For example, dieldrin formulations are extremely persistent, particularly the lacquers, and retain their effectiveness for many months. Chlordecone is formulated as a bait, whilst the organophosphorus and carbamate insecticides are usually applied as sprays. In choosing an insecticide it is important to remember that some strains of the German Cockroach (*Blatella germanica*) possess a high level of resistance to organochlorine insecticides and treatments with these compounds against such strains are doomed to failure. Mixtures can sometimes be usefully employed such as pyrethrins for rapid 'knock down' with BHC for persistence and kill, and in hot ducts and voids boric acid dust will remain active whereas other insecticides may break down and become ineffective in a very short time. The selection of the appropriate insecticide and formulation, and its application so that maximum effect is achieved, requires skill and experience, and is often best entrusted to professional pest control personnel. This is particularly so if the more toxic insecticides are to be used, when great care must be taken to prevent the accidental contamination of food and food preparation surfaces during application.

Ants

Ants are not known to be of any particular public health importance but they may be a nuisance in kitchens and other food premises on account of their desire to share the food of the human race. Much can be done to avoid attracting ants, by the most careful observance of cleanliness; even the smallest crumbs of waste food must be removed, and cracks and crevices which appear in walls and floors should be stopped up immediately. Two kinds of ant occur in buildings; garden-ants which nest outside but enter in search of food, and ants such as the Pharoah's ant, which nest in warm buildings. The best way to eliminate both types is to destroy the nest, and in the case of garden-ants this can be found and treated with boiling water or paraffin. When infestations are established indoors, however, it is a different matter. A war of attrition against the worker-ants can sometimes starve out the queen but losses in the ranks are so quickly made good that it is a lengthy process and the daily kill must be heavy. Insecticidal sprays and dusts containing chlordane, fenitrothion or dieldrin are reasonably effective, or insecticidal lacquer may be painted around cracks in walls or floors, over sills, near vents and on the underside of cupboard shelves. An alternative method of control is by poison bait using chlordecone incorporated in an attractive bait base. Pharaoh's ants have been reported to carry organisms of significance in human disease.

Wasps

Wasps can be a nuisance in food premises although there appears to be no evidence that they have been implicated in the spread of food infections. From mid-summer onwards the foraging workers are attracted by and feed on nectar and other sweet substances, but they will also take insects, fresh and decaying meat or fish to feed the grubs in the nest. Wasps seem to find their way into premises which would normally be regarded as fly-proof although they cannot penetrate mesh as fine as 3 mm ($\frac{1}{8}$ inch).

The workers may range half a mile or more from their nest and when an infestation occurs a search should be made for nests in the vicinity and steps taken to destroy them. This work is best carried out in the evening when most of the wasps are in the nest and drowsy, and it is a wise precaution for the operator to wear gauntlets and a bee-keeper's hood. When the nest is in a suitable position it can be soaked with a rapid 'knock-down' liquid insecticide and burnt or broken up. Equally quick results can be obtained for nests outside by pouring, or syringing, 1·4 to 2·8 decilitres ($\frac{1}{4}$ to $\frac{1}{2}$ pint) of carbon tetrachloride into the entrance hole of the nest and then plugging the hole.

A rather slower process is to place BHC, or derris powder dust at the entrance hole so that the insecticide is carried into the nest by the insects.

Where it is impossible to find or to deal with the nests, attractive baits set outside the premises will often intercept and divert wasps from the building. The bait may be jam, syrup, molasses, fermenting fruit or beer, mixed with enough water in a wide-mouthed jar to drown the insects. The addition of detergent (about a teaspoonful per 4·5 litres or 1 gallon) causes the trapped wasps to sink more quickly.

Safety Precautions

Unless care is taken, the use of any rodenticidal or insecticidal product in food premises can present risks to those who apply the materials, to those who work or dwell in the buildings and to those who consume the food that is present when the premises are treated.

Pesticides must always be applied strictly in accordance with the manufacturers instructions. Remember to read the label before use, and to carefully follow the advice which is given.

16

Legislation

(*The late L. KLUTH*)

Direct powers aimed to prevent the spread of food-borne infections are given by several statutes. The Public Health Act, 1936, requires the head of a household and any doctor attending a patient to report the occurrence of any case of notifiable disease, including typhoid fever, enteric fever or dysentery, to the medical officer of health; furthermore, it is an offence for a person suffering from a notifiable disease to carry on any business or occupation in which there is a risk of spreading the disease. More specifically, the Food and Drugs Act, 1955, requires a doctor who is aware of a case of food poisoning to report to the medical officer of health. In addition, any person working in food premises or a slaughterhouse who becomes aware that he is suffering from, or is carrying the agent of typhoid fever, paratyphoid fever, or any other salmonella infection or dysentery or any staphylococcal infection likely to cause food poisoning, must notify his employer, who in turn must notify the medical officer of health. Similar notification is required when any person having access to milk or receptacles in a dairy becomes aware that he or a member of his household is suffering from any notifiable disease (Food Hygiene (General) Regulations, 1970; Slaughterhouse (Hygiene) Regulations, 1958; Milk and Dairies (General) Regulations, 1959).

When information of this kind is received, the local authority may prohibit the employment of the person concerned in the handling of food and drink (Public Health (Infectious Diseases) Regulations, 1953; Milk and Dairies (General) Regulations, 1959).

When a medical officer of health suspects that a food is likely to cause food poisoning, and a sample is taken for examination, the further use of the food may be prohibited until the investigation is complete. Food proved to be unfit for human consumption may be seized (Food and Drugs Act, 1955). Other powers may be summarized as follows.

THE FOOD AND DRUGS ACT, 1955, seeks to protect the public against the sale of unsound food, and the adulteration and change of 'the nature, substance and quality' of food, and against false labelling and false advertisement. There are powers to punish wilful malpractice, secure sanitary conditions for storing and handling food to minimize the possibility of unintentional contamination, and prohibit the sale of food, either absolutely or until subjected to special processing—applicable to certain foods which are peculiarly liable to contamination at source. Furthermore, the Act:

1. Empowers authorized officers of a local authority to examine any food intended for human consumption, and where the food appears to be unsound to seize it and take it before a magistrate who decides whether it be fit or unfit.

Samples of food may be taken for chemical analysis and bacteriological examination, in order to assess firstly their nature, substance and quality and secondly the extent of bacterial contamination. Penalties exist within the Food and Drugs Act, 1955, regarding such offences.

2 (a) Restricts the use of premises for certain purposes, e.g. as dairies and slaughterhouses, for the manufacture of ice-cream and sausages, or for the preservation of food, to those which are acceptable on the grounds of hygiene and which are registered or licensed by local authorities.

(b) Gives power to the Secretary of State for Health and Social Security and to the Minister of Agriculture, Fisheries and Food, acting jointly, to make Regulations requiring the observance of sanitary and clean conditions and practices in storing, preparing and delivering food for human consumption (Food Hygiene (General) Regulations, 1970; Milk and Dairies (General) Regulations, 1959; Slaughterhouse (Hygiene) Regulations, 1958).

(c) Gives power to local authorities to make bye-laws relating to the hygiene of handling, wrapping and delivery of food.

3 (a) Forbids the sale, for human consumption, of any meat from knackers' yards, and of milk from any cow suffering from certain diseases, including tuberculosis and mastitis.

(b) Empowers the Secretaries of State to make Regulations, principally with the object of preventing the spread of bovine tuberculosis by milk, setting out the conditions under which milk may be sold under a special designation i.e. 'pasteurized', 'sterilized', Ultra Heat Treated as well as 'untreated', and also to specify by Order, areas in which no milk may be sold unless it carries a special designation (Milk (Special Designation) Regulations, 1963, as amended 1965).

(c) Empowers the Secretaries of State to make Regulations requiring the use of any process or treatment in the preparation of any food intended for sale for human consumption (e.g. the Ice-Cream (Heat treatment) Regulations, 1959, and the Liquid Egg (Pasteurization) Regulations, 1963).

MODEL BYE-LAWS on various hygienic measures indicate the form of clause which would be approved by the Secretary of State for adoption by local authorities; they were issued and taken up by many councils under an earlier Act. Such Bye-laws continue in force, and authorities may still make them. However, the Food Hygiene (General) Regulations, 1970, have to a large extent taken their place administratively, if for no other reason than that the penalties for contravention are greater under the Regulations.

It is not proposed, therefore, to go into any details of the requirements of bye-laws which add little or nothing to the Regulations.

THE FOOD HYGIENE (GENERAL) REGULATIONS, 1970, aim to secure a standard of construction and equipment in food premises and in home-based ships, where foods are handled, and of conduct by the food handlers so that the foodstuffs are protected from contamination. The requirements may be outlined as follows.

1. *Premises*

No food business shall be carried on at any insanitary premises, the condition, situation and construction of which is such that food is exposed to risk of contamination. The premises must be well lighted and ventilated, clean, free from accumulation of refuse and in good repair. There must be nothing about their situation or construction which could lead to the contamination of food and, in particular, sanitary conveniences must not be located in or approached directly from a food room. Similarly, food rooms may not be used as sleeping places or be directly entered from bedrooms. No fresh-air inlets or ventilation pipe connected with draining shall be situated in a food room.

2. *Sanitary facilities and other amenities*

A clean and wholesome water supply must be available, and there must be washing arrangements for food and equipment and for the use of the staff. Arrangements for hand washing must include basins, fixed where the employees can reach them quickly and easily, and provided with constant hot and cold (or blended) water, soap, nail brushes and clean towels.

For food and equipment there must be sinks or other washing equipment with constant hot and cold water, soap or detergent and means of drying. Where only fish, tripe, animal casings, fruit or vegetables are washed, cold water only need be supplied.

Sanitary conveniences must be well lit and ventilated; they must be kept clean and in good working order, with notices displayed requesting users to wash their hands.

There must be suitable accommodation for the outdoor clothing of employees, and an adequate supply of first-aid materials, including waterproof dressings.

3. *Equipment*

Articles of equipment in contact with food must be kept clean and in good repair. They must be made of non-absorbent material, and their form of construction should permit thorough cleansing and minimize risks of food contamination.

4. *Personal hygiene of food handlers*

Persons handling open food shall wear clean and washable overclothing, cover any open cut or abrasion with a waterproof dressing and refrain from spitting or smoking.

In general, he must protect food from contamination and, in particular when in the open, food must not be placed within 450 mm (18 inches) of the ground. It must not be carried in a dirty vehicle or container, or in a vehicle in which there is any live animal or poultry; it must not be wrapped in newspaper or other unclean material.

5. *Catering practice*

Where food premises are used for catering purposes, i.e. for the supply of food for immediate consumption, certain foods are required to be kept at temperatures either below 10 °C (50 °F) or not less than 62·8 °C (145 °F). They include meat, fish, gravy and imitation cream, foodstuffs prepared from or containing any of these substances or any egg, including dried or frozen whole egg, yolk or albumen, or milk including separated or skimmed, dried or condensed milk and cream.

The requirement does not, however, apply to any food actually exposed for sale, or to (a) bread, biscuits, cake or pastry in which egg or milk is used only prior to baking, (b) chocolate or sugar confectionery, (c) ice-cream to which Regulations requiring heat treatment apply, (d) food which is canned, bottled or otherwise preserved in an effectively closed container which remains unopened, (e) butter, margarine, lard, shortening, cooking fats or beef suet, (f) cheese, uncooked bacon, uncooked ham, dry pasta, dry pudding mixes, dry soup mixes or dry mixes for the preparation of beverages, (g) any unskinned rabbits or hares or unplucked game or poultry.

Most of the foods which are exempted from the Regulation are those which will not support the growth of micro-organisms because of factors such as low moisture content, high concentration of sugar, fat or salt, or because they are to be subsequently prepared and cooked.

A notable omission from the Food Hygiene Regulations concerns the storage of perishable foods exposed for sale. Cooked meatstuffs and sausages in particular should not be kept in food shops unless there are facilities to maintain them at a temperature of about 4 °C (39 °F); that is, cold storage should be provided both for window shows and retail use.

It is a common practice in certain retail shops whose main business is not concerned with catering to sell warmed pies from a heated display cabinet. Pies and pasties and spit-roasted chickens also may be kept warm, under conditions which would not satisfy requirements of the Regulations with regard to safe temperatures for storage of meat products.

Missing also from the Food Hygiene Regulations is reference to the fact that the food handler needs to protect himself against the foods he may be handling and in particular raw meat, offal and poultry. Conveniently placed wash-hand-basins should be available for frequent hand washing when preparing or serving raw meat cuts.

THE SLAUGHTERHOUSE (HYGIENE) REGULATIONS, 1958, as amended 1966, impose conditions of lay-out, structure and cleanliness, and of the conduct of employees, under which a local authority may license a slaughterhouse and without which a slaughterhouse may not be operated. Many of the requirements are similar to those of the Food Hygiene (General) Regulations, 1970, but there are points of special interest. Animals suspected of being diseased must be kept apart from the general lairage and slaughtered separately; separate accommodation must be provided for emptying the contents of stomachs and intestines, and also there must be separate locked accommodation for the retention, pending its early removal, of meat rejected as unfit. The hand may not be used for stirring blood intended for human consumption, and carcasses may not be inflated with the breath; knives, etc., must be cleansed and disinfected in boiling water or steam at the end of each working day, and immediately after use on a carcass suspected to be diseased. Cloths must not be used in a slaughterhouse for the purpose of wiping down any carcass or any offal.

Recognizing that the infection rate increases when animals are kept in lairs for 1 or 2 weeks awaiting slaughter, the amended Regulations limit the waiting period in such lairs to 72 hours except with the consent of an authorized officer to a longer stay. Lairs are required to be kept clean, and it is hoped that this will ensure the disinfection of lairs prior to the reception of each new group of animals.

THE MILK AND DAIRIES (GENERAL) REGULATIONS, 1959, provide for the veterinary inspection of cattle, and for standards of hygiene in the structure and cleanliness of dairy farms and dairies, and in operations carried on in such premises in order to qualify for compulsory registration.

Many of the requirements are similar to those of the Food Hygiene (General) Regulations, 1970, but those of special interest include the cleansing of the flanks, tail and udder of the cow, the hands of the milker and the milking stool before milking commences; foremilk must be inspected and discarded. Before removal to the milk room for cooling to 10 °C (50 °F) the milk must be kept covered; throughout the process of milking and preparation for distribution, appliances and vessels may be used only if, immediately beforehand, they have been thoroughly cleansed by being rinsed and washed, with and without detergent, and either scalded with boiling water or steam, or cleansed with an approved chemical agent. A list of approved chemical agents is given.

THE MILK (SPECIAL DESIGNATION) REGULATIONS, 1963, lay down that sealed containers must be labelled under licence 'untreated', 'pasteurized', or 'sterilized'.

The methods of treatment are prescribed as:

(a) pasteurization by holding the milk at temperatures between

62·8 °C (145 °F) and 65·6 °C (150 °F) for 30 minutes followed by immediate cooling to 10 °C (50 °F).

(b) pasteurization at 71·7 °C (161 °F) for 15 seconds, followed by immediate cooling to 10 °C (50 °F).

(a) and (b), the processed milk shall satisfy the methylene blue and phosphatase tests.

(c) 'sterilization', after filtration or clarification and homogenization, by heating to at least 100 °C (212 °F) in sealed bottles for an appropriate period to satisfy the turbidity test.

THE MILK (SPECIAL DESIGNATION) (AMENDMENT) REGULATIONS, 1965, permit the production and sale of milk, under licence from the local authority, as 'Ultra Heat Treated Milk'. To qualify for this description the milk must have been raised to and held at a temperature of 132 °C (270 °F) for 1 second in approved apparatus which automatically diverts any milk which does not reach the authorized temperature. Sterile containers must be filled aseptically, and sealed so as to be airtight, and any sample must satisfy a test in which fewer than 10 colonies of bacteria may develop from a loopful of milk in a prescribed medium incubated for 48 hours.

MILK (SPECIAL DESIGNATION) (AMENDMENT) REGULATIONS, 1972, came into operation on the 1st October 1972, and control the treatment by the direct application of steam in regard to 'Ultra Heat Treated' milk. It directs the methods to be employed in the injection and removal of steam, safeguards the milk content, temperature control and in the generation of steam lays down conditions for water treatment and sampling.

THE ICE-CREAM (HEAT TREATMENT, ETC.) REGULATIONS, 1959, require mixtures of ice-cream other than those from complete cold mixes already having received heat treatment, to be subjected, in apparatus appropriately designed for the purpose and fitted with suitable time/temperature recorders, to any of four alternative methods of heat treatment:

(a) pasteurization by holding at 65·6 °C (150 °F) for 30 minutes
(b) pasteurization by holding at 71·1 °C (160 °F) for 10 minutes
(c) pasteurization by holding at 79·4 °C (175 °F) for 15 seconds
(d) 'sterilization' by holding at 149 °C (300 °F) for 2 seconds.

The mixed ingredients may not be kept longer than 1 hour at a temperature higher than 7·2 °C (45 °F) before treatment, and after treating the temperature must be reduced to 7·2 °C (45 °F) within 1½ hours and so kept until frozen. If the temperature of the frozen ice-cream rises above −2·2 °C (28 °F) it must be retreated. There is an exception for mix held at 149 °C for 2 seconds: when transferred aseptically into sterile airtight containers it need not be reduced in temperature until required for freezing at the counter for 'soft ice-cream'.

THE LIQUID EGG (PASTEURIZATION) REGULATIONS, 1963, prohibit the use of untreated liquid whole egg as an ingredient in the preparation of food intended for sale for human consumption.

The pasteurization treatment requires the liquid egg to be held at 64·4 °C (148 °F) for 2½ minutes followed by immediate cooling to below 3·3 °C (38 °F), in apparatus appropriately designed for the purpose and fitted with a suitable time/temperature recorder.

The Regulations set out the method of sampling and examination by the alpha-amylase test, which the treated egg is required to satisfy.

THE PUBLIC HEALTH (SHELL-FISH) REGULATIONS, 1934 AND 1948, empower a local authority to prohibit the sale for human consumption of shell-fish, including mussels and cockles as well as oysters, from a laying within a district known to have produced shell-fish which have caused illness or likely to be dangerous to public health, unless subjected to an approved process of cleansing or sterilization.

THE MEAT (STERILIZATION) REGULATIONS, 1969, require that meat from knackers' yards, imported meat, and meat from any animal slaughtered in the United Kingdom intended for human consumption but unfit must be 'sterilized' before sale. Certain establishments such as zoos can obtain the unsterilized meat if it is transported in locked containers or vehicles.

'Sterilized' means treated by boiling or by steam under pressure until every piece of meat is cooked throughout, or dry-rendered, digested or solvent-processed into technical tallow, greases, glues, feeding meals or fertilizers.

THE IMPORTED FOOD REGULATIONS, 1968, define the authorities which enforce the Regulations. Any food commonly used for human consumption, which is imported, shall, until the contrary is proved, be presumed to have been imported for human consumption. The Port Health Authority may allow food to pass through the port without examination, provided notification is given to the local authority in whose area the food is to be delivered. The local authority then assumes the duties of a Port Health Authority with regard to the examination of the food and to the enforcement of the Regulations (this is due mainly to increased containerization, whereby food is imported in bulk in sealed containers).

The importation of food unfit for human consumption is prohibited. An authorized officer may at all reasonable times examine food which has been imported for sale for human consumption, and where it is seen to be unfit, he may seize it and take action under Section 8 of the Food and Drugs Act, 1955. Samples of food may be taken for analysis, and where special examination is necessary the food may be held for periods up to 6 days pending results of the examination. Meat and meat products require to be accompanied by an official certificate from the country of origin.

Additional needs

Legislation cannot be introduced in advance of the results of informed opinion in technical investigation and, although there are instances of control being rapidly applied to new and undesirable practices, e.g. the Meat (Treatment) Regulations, 1964—which prohibit the use of certain additives to meat—measures for the prevention of bacteriological food poisoning have been slow to come. Dried egg was implicated as a vehicle of infection in 1940 and liquid whole egg in 1955, yet the pasteurization of this product was not made compulsory until 1963. The delay was due partly to industrial and commercial difficulties and partly to difficulties in perfecting the alpha-amylase test as a means to control the efficiency of pasteurization at the recommended temperature and time.

The widest implications of the failure to maintain a disease-free animal population are perhaps insufficiently appreciated. Although there has been success in the eradication of tuberculosis from dairy cattle, and measures can be readily instituted to contain outbreaks of animal diseases which are notifiable, there is still a substantial reservoir of, for example, salmonellae in farm animals including cattle, pigs, and poultry; the control of such infection is under review. A scheme for the eradication of brucellosis is now in operation and will gradually involve the whole of the country.

One serious impediment to the establishment of salmonella-free stock is the persistent use of contaminated feeding stuffs. Although a high proportion of informal samples of bone, meat and fish meals from a wide variety of countries indicate the presence of salmonellae, these animal feeding stuffs and fertilizers are not yet subject to nationally effective bacteriological control either at the ports or in places of manufacture or elsewhere. The evidence against these products is sufficient to merit an extension of the powers of local authorities under the Fertilizers and Feeding Stuffs Act, 1968. Significant bacterial contamination should be added to the physical and chemical impurities which can be dealt with as deleterious substances in feeding stuffs under the Act, and provision made for such materials to undergo an approved treatment.

Other orders such as the Waste Food (Disease of Animals Act (Waste Foods)) Order, 1957, may be extended to include imported and home-produced feeding meals of animal origin. Condemned meat must now be removed in locked vans and labelled as such, and processed for inedible use or 'sterilized' for animal feeding.

Whilst foci of infection remain in farm animals, the law should require greater precautions against cross-infection and cross-contamination. The sale and showing and even movement of known symptomless excretors should be forbidden. The suggestion that symptomless excreters of salmonellae should be notifiable is now under consideration. It has been shown that animals transported long distances suffer stress causing higher rates of salmonella excretion. The transport of calves and their introduction while excreting *Salmonella typhimurium* into farms engaged in the intensive rearing of young cattle for beef needs control. At present the welfare of the animals is covered by the Transit of Calves Order, 1963, under the Diseases of Animals Act, 1950, but the public health aspect is not considered.

The hazard of salmonellae in calves is reduced if they are reared for 2 to 3 weeks on the farm where they are born.

The widespread use of antibiotics in animal feeds and for treatment was held responsible for the rapid increase in antibiotic-resistant strains of *S. typhimurium*. The veterinary and industrial use of antibiotics is now controlled by the Therapeutic Substances Act, 1956.

So much of the spread of infection is concerned with the transfer of organisms between animals and man via foodstuffs that the epidemiological investigation not only of outbreaks but of the spread of salmonellae in general involves the combined efforts of medical, veterinary and public health workers together with food technologists.

Now that local authorities are required to inspect all meat for human consumption from slaughterhouses, the extension of this duty to poultry killed for the table is in force for exports and under consideration for poultry intended for home consumption. The development of systems of line slaughter facilitates inspection, and thus the killing of a high proportion of the birds which make up the 570,000 tons (579,142·8 tonnes) of poultry carcasses sold annually could, by a system of registration, be restricted to places where proper inspection is practicable.

It seems unrealistic that equipment which comes into contact with food should be required (or permitted) to undergo different methods of cleansing in dairies, slaughterhouses, and other food premises. If approved chemical cleansing agents are acceptable for milk vessels and plants (and there are some ninety brand names officially sanctioned), there seems to be no reason for restricting the methods of treating slaughterhouse equipment to boiling water and steam. Indeed, with means so readily available why do not the Food Hygiene Regulations require the disinfection of food equipment in food preparation premises generally and also indicate the methods or substances which should be used?

Certain foods such as bulked liquid or frozen whole eggs which are especially liable to be contaminated at source are already required to receive some form of treatment to render them safe, but it may well be thought that such protective measures should be prescribed to all bulked egg products. A heat-treatment process is now under investigation for liquid egg white and should be required as standard practice when it is proved to be practicable. In the case of milk, the original purpose of pasteurization (as a measure against tuberculosis) has lapsed with the achievement of tubercle-free dairy herds, but the process continues to be of immense public health value since milk is liable to infection at source from Brucella, staphylococci, salmonellae and numerous other organisms. It is unlikely that the approved method of heat treatment will ever be abandoned for the great bulk of supplies, but raw milk may still be sold for manufacturing purposes, including cheese, and retailed under the designation 'untreated'. These two outlets for untreated milk are breaches of the national defences against milk-borne diseases other than tuberculosis.

Under the Milk and Dairies (General) Regulations, 1959, milk is defined to include cream. Anyone dealing in fresh cream must, therefore, be registered along with the premises. Under the Milk (Special Designation) Regulations, 1963, cream is excluded. The former regulations are administered by the local authority and environmental and health standards in the handling of fresh cream are laid down. The 1963 Regulations are administered by county councils and county boroughs and deal with licensing and testing of milk only. One writer suggests that as a result milk dairies receive far more attention than cream dairies, even when a milk dairy houses a cream section. The feeling in the trade is that if the government does not consider the production and selling of fresh cream important enough to warrant licensing, there cannot be any need to give the production of fresh cream special attention.

The routine sampling of fresh cream has shown that many samples are heavily contaminated, thus recommendations with regard to treatment and a grading scheme, already suggested by the Public Health Laboratory Service and similar to that used for ice-cream, are required.

After the local government reorganization on 1 April 1974 the former divisions into counties, boroughs, urban and rural districts disappeared, although in some instances the names are retained for reasons of sentiment. The operational unit is now the District. Within this unit, some of the statutory powers formerly exercised by the medical officer of health are exercised by a medically qualified 'proper officer', who is generally a community physician seconded to the local government District by the relevant health District of the National Health Service. Other statutory powers are exercised by an environmental health officer acting in his own right as a 'proper officer' of local government.

The preceding and the following chapter should be read in the light of this new situation. Policies should now be uniform within the new Districts. The new 'proper officers' can be contacted through the local health departments.

17
Education

The prevention of food poisoning is the concern of all those who provide foodstuffs not only for human consumption but for animal consumption also. The engineers who design equipment and the architects responsible for planning kitchens, manufacturing establishments, slaughterhouses, markets and farms also have an important part to play for they can help to control the spread of infection.

All these groups of people, therefore, from the architects, farmers and plant engineers to every food handler concerned with manufacture, retail trade or kitchen, should receive information on the causes of food poisoning and on the sources of the various bacterial agents and means of control. In this respect the word 'control' covers protection of both man and animal against invasion by disease-bearing groups of bacteria, prevention of their transmission to foodstuffs by living agents and equipment, and prevention of their multiplication in foodstuffs.

The necessity for this teaching may be justified by a summary of the latest annual figures for food poisoning in England and Wales available every year from the Chief Medical Officer of the Department of Health and Social Security (DHSS), and Public Health Laboratory Service. In 1970, for example, there were 6,107 incidents and each incident may be one case only or hundreds of cases. It is estimated that 9,000 or more cases of food poisoning occur each year but there may be many others which are not reported. There is legislation to ensure that the disease of food poisoning is notified to the DHSS but many incidents are not reported to the doctor and thus the information will not reach the medical officer of health, public health laboratory and DHSS. A large number of single incidents, regarded as sporadic cases, may be part of one large outbreak from a contaminated foodstuff distributed widely over the country, but unrecognized as a source of danger.

The outbreaks most commonly notified are those which occur in institutions feeding large numbers of people such as schools, hospitals and factories where faults in the daily feeding of the same groups of people cannot fail to be observed. The same faults

239

causing illness in persons making chance visits to hotels, cafés and restaurants, or in travellers may pass unnoticed.

Meat and poultry in their various forms are the foods most commonly implicated and they are responsible yearly for more than half the notified incidents of food poisoning.

An appreciable reduction in the incidence of salmonella food poisoning may be achieved ultimately by controlling the animal sources. To control staphylococcal food poisoning there must be strict attention to techniques used for the manipulation of cooked foods such as meats and custard type dishes. Prevention of *Clostridium welchii* food poisoning is concerned with care in cooling and cold storage of bulks of meat and poultry. In all instances cold storage of cooked food is important as well as environmental design and cleanliness. Provision of good conditions is the responsibility of the management, in whom, as well as in the food handlers, rests the care of the food they provide and sell.

Widespread and persistent instruction is needed to implant the necessity for correct methods in the minds of responsible people. Groups receptive to information about the causes of food-borne disease and its prevention may vary from girls and boys in schools to the adult staff, including managers and supervisors as well as employees, of the catering and food industries. Medical officers of health and health inspectors require the latest knowledge for teaching purposes. There will be many different levels of perception, experience and purpose, and a speaker must select information fitted to the needs of each audience. It is probably better to err by giving too many facts rather than to underestimate the lively interest of non-technical groups.

Suggested lecture headings for various groups of people are given in Appendix A to this chapter.

Schools

Children may be taught how infection spreads and they are usually interested in the subject.

Hygienic habits are not instinctive; they need to be implanted early to persist in later life. The instruction necessary for their acquisition may not always be given in the home; the responsibility, therefore, falls partly on the school. In those schools teaching domestic science as a routine part of the curriculum, elementary bacteriology and its application to the prevention of food contamination can be conveniently taught and demonstrated practically during cookery lessons. Useful supplementary education can be given to schools by the local public health departments; this is already carried out in some boroughs by the health inspectors and health education officers.

Practical demonstrations can be given with petri dish cultures of the growth of bacteria from the hands, nose, throat and bowel and showing the vastly increased bacterial flora on the hands after touching raw meat and poultry and other foods. The effect of washing the hands can be shown. Cultures from damp swabs rubbed over various surfaces, utensils and equipment will illustrate the differences in bacterial cleanliness between surfaces of wood and the more impervious materials. Also, foodstuffs can be cultured as purchased and after storage in the kitchen and in the refrigerator in order to demonstrate the effect of different storage temperatures on the numbers of bacteria in foods.

When food hygiene demonstrations are available, parties from schools should be taken round the various exhibits with an explanatory running commentary. Competitions may be held between schools on the composition of a picture showing some particular aspect of food hygiene and the winning picture displayed at the exhibition. The interest aroused by such competitions is likely to be widespread, not only amongst school friends of the entrant but in home circles.

The school meals service has grown from the days of soup, bread and cake to a thriving business which, in England alone, provides 5 million children each day with varied two-course meals. This midday meal is subsidized by the government, and in certain instances is provided free of charge. The country is divided into approximately 163 local authorities, each with its own school meals organizer and assistants. In a large kitchen the staff includes the supervisor or cook supervisor, the cook, the assistant cook and helpers. All new schools are provided with their own kitchen, and new kitchens are being built for existing schools as far as possible. A central kitchen may produce as many as 700 or more meals a day for 13 or 14 schools; it may also provide meals for old people in the area.

Members of the staff for the school meals service are generally trained to a high degree of efficiency. In the North Riding of Yorkshire they attend in-service training courses on hygiene and nutrition at their residential College for Further Education. In addition, staff are encouraged to study for the City and Guilds qualifications at the colleges of further education or to attend locally arranged courses which could include certificate courses on the hygienic handling of food.

Lectures on food hygiene to groups of organizers and cooks are most rewarding and the results may be seen in the desire for improved methods and equipment. Domestic science teachers in schools and hospitals also request talks, sometimes after the usual teaching hours and as part of week-end training courses.

Hospitals

Each regional board has an officer responsible for all training schemes; they arrange courses for various classes of hospital officers within their region, either at their own centre or in conjunction with local technical colleges. Several regions give supervisory courses for catering personnel; the subject of food safety and quality is sometimes included. The teaching of hygiene in hospitals is considered in the Department of Health Circular H.M. (64) 34.

In courses for potential catering officers, food hygiene is taught during the practical period before trainees enter their formal year of administration. Basic training for catering officers and supervisors is provided by universities and technical colleges.

For many years the Staff College for Hospital Caterers organized by King Edward's Hospital Fund for London provided courses for all ranks of hospital catering staff; lectures were given on hygiene, food organization, diet and the preparation and sources of food.

Restaurants, hotels and factories and food handlers in retail shops

Special curricula reaching degree level in technical colleges are available for students wanting responsible work in the catering industry as well as in hospitals. University and independent colleges also give training in domestic science which includes food hygiene. There are correspondence courses available also. The Hotel and Catering Institute examinations held yearly provide papers on food hygiene and nutrition.

There are two methods used separately or in conjunction with each other for the teaching of food handlers in commercial eating establishments and shops. The first seeks to gather together the managers, supervisors and other key personnel for a series of lectures. Three or four talks may be given at weekly or shorter intervals. The provision of comprehensive lecture notes will help the dissemination of information to employees, or better still a similar course can be given to all kitchen staff.

For large catering establishments and multiple stores this method can be used within the shop or store. For school kitchens it may be convenient to arrange a meeting at one particular centre, under the control of the local authority. The owners and assistants of small establishments including shops, cafés, snack-bars and portable food vans may be attracted to these meetings; otherwise, special courses of lectures should be given for them. Public lecture demonstrations and exhibitions with films may attract a wider audience, discussions should be encouraged and free literature available.

The second method is to go out to people rather than to invite them to a centre. This may be arranged fairly readily in large or small establishments by the resident medical officer and local health inspectors or other suitably qualified persons. Demonstration material may be taken to various departments and talks given on the spot to small groups of staff within the kitchen or shop. Public talks and exhibitions should be followed by visits and further discussions.

The Catering Trade Working Party, in the Report published in 1951, stated that 'no large scale and lasting improvement in the hygienic conditions of catering establishments can be brought about unless informed public opinion demands it. We would stress the word "informed" because many people, while appreciating generally the value of cleanliness, have little knowledge of the real risks attendant on particular faulty practices. The dissemination of knowledge of the principles underlying food hygiene should, therefore, be carried out by practical means.' There has been much improvement in the standard of kitchens since that was written but the hazards leading to food poisoning are still not always fully understood by those who must avoid them.

PROVISION OF INFORMATION

Information on food hygiene is available from many sources, but much of the responsibility for assimilating facts is assumed nationally by the medical officers of health, health inspectors, health education officers and other public health workers. In many European countries and in the USA the veterinary officer takes a prominent part also. The health inspector is the link between the medical officer of health and the food trader, restaurant and canteen supervisor and other food handlers in his area; his district work keeps him constantly in touch with a wide variety of food workers. The success of any drive to establish and maintain better conditions and techniques amongst food handlers will depend largely on his efforts. Health inspectors trained by local authorities are sometimes employed by the food and catering industries to help both in the education of food handlers and in the maintenance of high standards of hygiene in food production and preparation.

In 1972 a committee of experienced health inspectors reported that lack of administrative action in certain areas resulted in malpractice. They recommended the registration of all catering premises and stressed the need for inspection by local authorities of kitchens in establishments, such as hospitals and other 'Crown Property', now exempt from local authority care.

Administrative experts of the Department of Health and Social Security are available for advice and lectures on legislation and Codes of Practice; pictorial charts, pamphlets and other display material may be obtained from the education section of the DHSS. The Ministry of Agriculture, Fisheries and Food provides a similar service for the veterinary profession and industry.

The Public Health Laboratory Service in England and Wales is active in the field of education on matters relating to the prevention of bacterial and viral diseases. Amongst the many functions of these laboratories, scattered throughout the country, are the examination of foodstuffs associated with outbreaks of food poisoning and the investigation of the sources and means of spread of the bacterial agents responsible.

Regular samples of home-produced and imported food, as well as milk, water and ice-cream are examined for sanitary control. Surveillance studies and research are carried out on foods known to be public health hazards and suspected to spread bacterial agents in manufacturing establishments, shops and kitchens. The zoonotic illnesses due to bacteria shared between man and animals and which cause both to suffer are investigated jointly with the veterinary profession.

The results of epidemiological studies on outbreaks of food poisoning and the conclusions reached on the spread of food-poisoning organisms from humans, animal and food sources in relation to the prevention of food-borne disease are communicated to others. Talks are given to medical officers of health, health inspectors, veterinary officers and other members of local government departments, domestic science teachers, scholars and students in school and colleges, school and university meals staff, hospital staff, women's organizations and industrial and national concerns. Contributions to books and journals distribute information nationally and internationally.

Agricultural Research Council Laboratories, such as those of the Meat Research Institute, Food Research Institute, and Poultry Research Station, the food research laboratories of the manufacturing and baking industries and of the Atomic Energy Authority and other independent laboratories are continually checking and investigating means of preventing food spoilage, as well as the contamination and build-up of pathogenic organisms in food.

Independent organizations active in the field of food hygiene education include the Central Council for Health Education, the Associations of Industrial Management, Industrial Welfare and St. John Ambulance, the Red Cross, Women's Institutes, Women's Royal Voluntary Service, the organizations for Housecraft, and Scientific Management in the Home and church groups.

Short courses on food hygiene are given by the Royal Society of Health and the Institute of Public Health and Hygiene. Booklets are available for teaching purposes, such as *Hygienic Food Handling* available from the St. John Ambulance Association which is also willing to provide lecture courses on food hygiene. A simplified version of the Food Hygiene (1970) Regulations is published by the Central Council for Health Education. Journals and magazines of various associations such as *Hotel and Restaurant Management, The Hotel Catering and Institutional Management Association Journal, Environmental Health, Royal Society of Health Journal, Nutrition and Food Science*, as well as the more general periodicals, particularly those specializing in domestic subjects, provide many opportunities for publicizing information.

The King Edward's Hospital Fund for London has already been mentioned in relation to the Staff College for Hospital Caterers; in addition, for many years it has supported an excellent Hospital Catering Advisory Service providing a centre with model kitchens and equipment and facilities for lectures. This service instituted trials of new feeding systems for hospitals; for example, the use of frozen cooked meals and frozen prepared single items issued from central kitchens or food manufacturers, and methods to thaw and reheat including hot air circulation and microwave ovens. The Ganymede 'Heatstor', Helitherm, Finessa and Stellex systems for meal distribution operate with conventional cookery and incorporate a centralized tray service with special trays and trolleys. As trays move along on a conveyor belt, food items are added to them. There are bulk food *bain maries* and automatic dispensers for plates, plate covers and trays.

The principal difference between the Stellex and Ganymede systems is in the method of keeping food hot. In the Stellex system, electrically heated elements remain *in situ* in the trolley, the dinner and sweet plates resting directly on them. The trolleys then convey the trays to the wards. Another difference is that with the Stellex system soup is sent in bulk and served by the ward sister. Sauces and gravies may also be added at the time of presentation to the patient.

Finessa is similar to Ganymede 'Heatstor' but Helitherm retains heat in the food by insulated glass fibre trays.

The time for meal assembly and presentation to the patient is said to be 5 to 10 minutes, allowing another 15 to 20 minutes for actual consumption of the meal, giving a total of 20 to 30 minutes from time of assembly of the food on the tray to final consumption by the patient.

The Regethermic system is based on the precooking, plating and rapid chilling of meals up to 48 hours in advance of service. The cooked food is plated and cooled to a temperature below 5 °C (38 °F) in less than 45 minutes and stored at this temperature. When convenient the meals are sent to the wards where they are kept in a refrigerator. When the meals are required they are placed in a Regethermic regeneration or reheat oven which raises the temperature to 85 °C (180 °F) within 10 minutes. The fresh hot appearance of the food is appreciated by the patients. The Peripheral Finishing kitchen works on the basis of last minute cooking of food which depreciates in palatability or nutritionally.

Reports on these various systems are available and are published by the King Edward's Hospital Fund for London.

The Central Office of Information, various industries, and overseas teaching laboratories such as the Center for Disease Control, Atlanta, and universities in the USA such as those in Indiana and Minnesota produce films, slides and bulletins. The larger catering firms, food industrialists, shipping firms and airways carry far afield the principles of food hygiene as taught in the United Kingdom.

Many commercial firms engaged in the manufacture of foods, equipment and detergents willingly provide exhibits for educational purposes.

The popularity of summer schools, week-end and other refresher courses is growing; the range of subjects is large and they serve a useful purpose in the field of food hygiene for domestic science teachers, hospital and school catering staff and other persons concerned with general health education as well as with the production of safe food.

Television and broadcast programmes for both adults and schools have a wide appeal. Newspaper reports of outbreaks of food poisoning should be as accurate as possible, thus the press should be given full information including sponsored notes on the faults and reasons which lead to outbreaks, the method of spread of infection and how it can be prevented.

Clean Food Guilds

The first Clean Food Guild for the food trade was initiated at Guildford in 1947. Other towns and boroughs followed with similar guilds. Some of these, including the Guildford Guild, are still flourishing and others are no longer in existence, but new ones are starting. There are various activities included in these organizations. Usually there is a Code of Practice for food traders and catering food handlers. Instruction is given at a series of lectures on food and kitchen hygiene. Adherence to the compulsory attendance leads to a certificate; in some places a simple examination may be held. When the hygienic arrangements and methods employed in catering establishments or other food shops comply with the recommendations laid down in the codes of practice, and when each member of the staff has been issued with a certificate for attendance at the lectures, then a certificate of merit is awarded to the establishment. This certificate may be displayed in the shop window. One advantage of voluntarily accepted codes of practice is that the requirements of a statutory nature may be expressed in practical terms; for example, the cleanliness of utensils required by the Act may be secured, let us say, by the use of a disinfecting rinse in water at $82 \cdot 2 \,^{\circ}\mathrm{C}$ ($180\,^{\circ}\mathrm{F}$) after the utensils have been washed.

The guild system has been criticized because establishments awarded a certificate of merit do not always maintain their high standard. This might be overcome by a grading system based on points given for good equipment and hygienic methods. Down-grading to the point of removal of the certificate may result in greater efforts to maintain proficiency. The whole scheme is dependent on the constant watchfulness, persistence and en-couragement of the local authority health officers. Good liaison and relationship between the officers of the public health depart-ments and local food handlers may be encouraged by social meetings for informal talks and discussions. Mutual confidence between members of these groups, whether local authority health officers or food handlers, will improve standards faster than policing tactics.

Aids to teaching food hygiene

Semi-technical lectures to non-technical audiences are best illustrated with the aid of visual demonstrations. Film-strips may be shown and accompanied by a running commentary; a large multiple store engaged in extensive work amongst its food-handling employees has used a film-strip together with the recorded voice of a commentator. A combined unit has been devised containing film-strip, projector and gramophone recorder, so that film-strips and sound discs can be sent around the country and used when no experienced lecturer on the subject is available.

Thirty-five mm coloured slides and other aids to projection are valuable assets even to more technical lectures. Charts and tables may be used to show the rise in any particular type of food poison-ing, the increase in food poisoning during the summer months and the predominance of meats and poultry as food vehicles in gastroenteritis. Tables may be used to show recent laboratory findings on food sources of salmonellae. When methods have been found to render the foods safe by pasteurization or irradiation, for example, these can be shown by tables and charts also.

Amateur photography can be used to illustrate good and bad practices in the kitchen. Environmental factors such as design of surface structure, equipment, storage, washing-up procedures and garbage disposal may show clearly in picture form facts that may be difficult to express in words. Large charts and posters may be photographed and shown on the screen when travelling makes transportation of equipment difficult.

Films also illustrate in a life-like manner points which may be unconvincing by the spoken word. They should be preceded by an explanatory talk on the sources of food-poisoning organisms, methods of spread, conditions which encourage multiplication in foods and methods of prevention. A preparatory talk will help the audience to appreciate more fully faults illustrated in the film. 'Another Case of Food Poisoning' is admirable for teaching purposes. It was produced by the Central Office of Information and sponsored by the Ministry of Health (now Department of Health and Social Security) in collaboration with the Central Council for Health Education (now the Health Education Council), the Ministry of Food (now Ministry of Agriculture, Fisheries and Food) and the British Tourist and Holiday Board (now the British Tourist Authority). Two other noteworthy films are the Gas Council's 'Most Precious Gift', which illustrates the use of water by the example of a food poisoning story, and 'Food without Fear', produced by Diversey Products. The first half of this latter film shows the various ways of spread of contaminating bacteria in a kitchen and also gives a graphic description of the effect of temperature on growth. 'Most Precious Gift' gives advertising material also but this can be explained in the preparatory talk. Another film, by Bowater Scott, advertises paper towels for the prevention of cross-infection. A list of publications and teaching aids, including films and filmstrips, is available from the Health Education Council. There are excellent films prepared in the USA; for example, 'Epidemiology of Salmonellosis', which cites statistics on food poisoning and describes the animal sources of salmonellae and their spread by means of food. A list of films is available from the Center for Disease Control, Atlanta, Georgia.

Illustrations in the form of charts, diagrams, posters and photographs may be usefully displayed in a lecture room for the interest of those arriving early, or for those who are prepared to stay after the talk. Some charts and posters will give factual information; for example, graphs which show the rise or fall in incidence of food poisoning in England and Wales during the current years. Others may indicate, in a simple diagrammatic form, the reservoirs of infection and the way in which the bacterial agents spread. The critical temperatures of storage for foods and the rates of multiplication of bacteria in foods under different conditions of storage may be illustrated also. Simple pictorial stories in colour of actual outbreaks of food poisoning with short explanatory headings have proved to be popular both for use in lecture demonstrations and for exhibitions; they can be photographed for slides. Examples of these story charts are given in Chapter 6. A poster may serve to illustrate a single fact in a straightforward serious manner, or factual evidence may be presented in a humorous way by a famous cartoonist; the late Fougasse designed many posters for the Central Council for Health Education (now the Health Education Council).

Photographs to illustrate well designed kitchens with emphasis on structure and procedures for cleaning and storage should be mounted on stiff card; they may be issued singly or in series illustrating a certain sequence of events.

Bacterial cultures on various agar media in petri dishes may be shown by means of an illuminated viewing box. Such plate cultures can be used to demonstrate bacterial colonies from fingers rubbed lightly on the surface of the media. Comparative culture plates will show the effect of touching food and the efficacy or otherwise of washing the hands, the growth from clean and dirty handkerchiefs, kitchen cloths, towels and surfaces. Hairs and flies may be placed on agar plates also. Colonies of bacteria may be grown from imperfectly washed utensils. Portions of food may be cultured in agar media to illustrate bacteriologically clean and dirty food, and the effect of refrigeration on the prevention of bacterial growth. In addition, pure cultures of food-poisoning bacteria can be used to show the colonial appearance of salmonella, staphylococci, *Clostridium welchii*, *Bacillus cereus* and other organisms. There has been a great demand for plates of this type to illustrate, in a practical way, the facts that have been expressed in a talk.

Swabs may be taken from plates, cups, spoons, forks, table tops, floor, paper money, handkerchiefs, cloths and other objects frequently used, and suggested by members of the class. Various kinds of raw and cooked foods can be cultured to demonstrate the bacterial content as purchased and after storage. The contamination of fingers by food, such as raw meats and poultry, can be shown by the growth of bacteria on comparative plates before and after touching the food; the hands should be washed and recultured.

The ease of spread of infection may be demonstrated with the help of a dye. The handle of a saucepan or other utensil is coated with Vaseline petroleum jelly or similar sticky material containing a red dye. A member of the class is asked to grasp the handle, then to pick up one or two other utensils, walk in and out of a room, turning the door handle with the contaminated hand, turn a tap, wash the hands, turn off the tap and wipe the hands. When the surfaces touched by the 'contaminated' hand are wiped with a piece of white cotton wool, the red dye is easily seen on the cotton wool and also on the towel used after retouching the 'contaminated' tap.

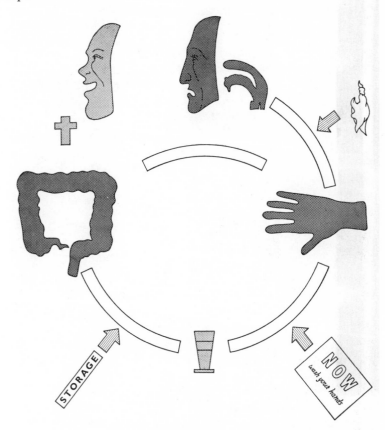

FIG. 54.   Flannelgraph showing chain of infection

Open petri dishes containing culture media may be exposed in various parts of the room during the course of a lecture to demonstrate the presence of bacteria in dust and droplet particles.

The flannelgraph is a useful method to focus attention on headings, important facts, pictorial diagrams and coloured sketches emphasizing points from a lecture. Once prepared, the printed and pictorial messages can be used many times and save the labour of blackboard work before and during a talk. A flannelgraph

board can be improvised with a large piece of flannel, felt or lint
pinned on to a blackboard. Alternatively, a suitable piece of
plywood can be covered with flannel, felt or lint; it is light

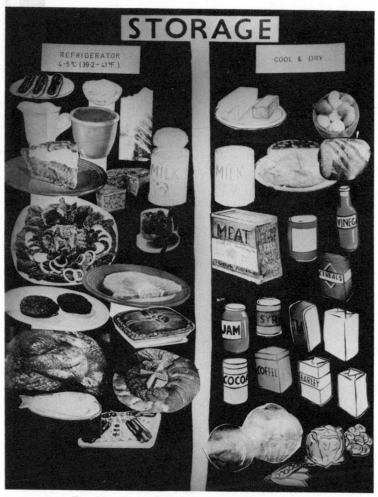

FIG. 55.   Flannelgraph showing correct storage

and can be carried easily from place to place. The printed headings, diagrams and pictures drawn on moderately stiff paper
are backed with flannel or lint; the material may be stuck over the
whole of the back area of the cut-out or applied in small strips or

discs. Flannel and lint adhere to each other and it is necessary only to place the prepared data firmly on the covered wood or blackboard (Figs. 54 and 55). To provide a similar method of display, small magnets can be stuck to the back of the printed and drawn material which adhere to a special type of metal sheet instead of the covered blackboard or plywood.

Overhead projection, from apparatus which throws on to a screen or wall writing or diagrams on micro-sheets, is helpful to illustrate a lecture as it proceeds. The written notes or diagrams may be prepared beforehand; last-minute thoughts are quickly transferred to

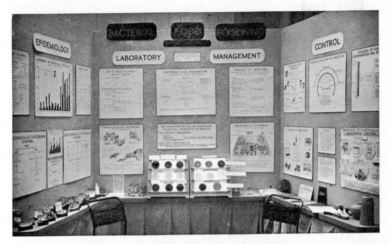

FIG. 56.   Display unit

the sheets. A similar system provides coated glass slides which may be etched with a sharp instrument and shown through a lantern. Special paint may be used for colour writing on glass slides or the micro-sheets.

During a lecture session it is possible to use the flannelgraph or overhead projection, lantern slides and also an illuminated viewing box to display culture plates; diagrams, charts and photographs may be displayed around the room for the members of the class or audience to study at their leisure.

Food hygiene sessions with lectures and exhibition material have been held in the dining-rooms of school canteens; the kitchen is used for demonstrations and discussion.

Investigations into the causes of bacterial food poisoning continually reveal new facts and the information should be passed on

TABLE 16. Sources and control of food-poisoning bacteria

Source	Public Health control	Laboratory control
	Salmonella	
Animal		
stool, coat, hooves, paws	Rearing methods Feeding stuffs Farm hygiene Slaughterhouse hygiene	Diagnostic media for stool samples, swabs and food Bacteriological counts on foods and feeds Biochemical tests Serological and bacteriophage typing
Foodstuffs (animal origin)		
meat and poultry feeding stuffs for animals, egg products, raw milk	Hygiene of production Treatment to render safe Storage	
Environment of food preparation	Cleanliness of equipment, utensils and surfaces	
Water for drinking and preparation of food	Treatment by filtration and chlorination	
Human stool, hand	Care in handling foods Avoidance of cross-contamination from raw to cooked food Personal hygiene	
	Staphylococcus	
Human nose, throat, hand, skin and lesions	Care in handling foods Storage of cooked foods Personal hygiene and habits	Diagnostic media for swabs and food Bacteriological counts on food
Animal cow, goat	Care of mastitis	Coagulase test Bacteriophage and serological typing
Foodstuffs (dairy) milk, cheese, cream	Hygiene of milk production Heat treatment of milk intended for drinking and for cream and cheese	Enterotoxin detection by gel diffusion techniques
	Clostridium welchii	
Foodstuff meat and poultry, dehydrated foods	Cooking and cooling techniques Storage of cooked food	Diagnostic media for stool samples and food Bacteriological counts on food

TABLE 16. (cont.) Sources and control of food-poisoning bacteria

Source	Public Health control	Laboratory control
	Clostridium welchii (cont.)	
Environment	Cleanliness of equipment	*Cl. welchii* counts on stools
of food preparation	and surfaces	Serological typing
(food and dust)		
Human		
stool		
Animal		
stools and dust		
	Clostridium botulinum	
Soil and mud		Toxin identification
Fish	Processing and cooking	(neutralization tests in
Foodstuff		mice)
fish, meat and		Diagnostic media
vegetables		
	Bacillus cereus	
Foodstuff (cereals)	Storage after cooking	Diagnostic media
dust, soil	Cleanliness of	Bacteriological counts on
	environment	food
		Serological typing
	Vibrio parahaemolyticus	
Seafoods	Warning against eating	Diagnostic media
	raw fish and other	Bacteriological counts on
	seafoods	food
	Avoidance of cross-	Serological typing
	contamination from	
	raw to cooked seafood	
	Other organisms, e.g. streptococci	
Human	General care of food	Diagnostic media
Animal	and storage	Bacteriological counts on
Foodstuff		food
		Serological typing

(Modified from Herschdoerfer, S. M., 1967, *Quality Control in the Food Industry*, Vol. 1. Academic Press, New York and London.)

to food handlers so that they can be taught to play their part in breaking the chains of infection which give rise to one outbreak after another. Education about food poisoning and its prevention is essential if this intestinal disease is to be brought under control. The subject interests most people because it affects everyone.

Teaching requires a knowledge of the statistical facts about food poisoning and also familiarity with the sources and habits and general behaviour in food of the various organisms responsible for food-borne illness.

A set of rules to control one organism may do little to stop the activities of another. For example, emphasis on personal hygiene alone may reduce the incidence of staphylococcal food poisoning but it will do little to prevent salmonellosis and nothing to stop *Clostridium welchii* food poisoning. Even the strictest rules of personal hygiene will not prevent outbreaks when large quantities of contaminated raw foods are handled by people unaware of the presence of salmonellae in the food and in their immediate environmental surroundings. The onus of producing salmonella-free foods goes far back in the chain of production and it should not be the responsibility of those who handle food after distribution at the

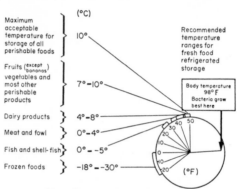

FIG. 57. Cold storage for foods

retail and consumer end. Recommendations to help the retail and consumer trade are essential but, by right, they should expect to be given safe food.

All the usual precautions against *Cl. welchii* and *B. cereus* food poisoning will fail unless it is understood that the spores of these organisms can survive cooking and must be prevented from growing out into active bacilli by rapid cooling and cold storage of meat and poultry dishes (*Cl. welchii*) and rice (*B. cereus*) if the foods are not to be eaten freshly cooked and hot. Perhaps the greatest of all the measures against food poisoning is the prevention of bacterial growth in foods after cooking by attention to cooling times and cold storage.

It is possible to teach the general principles which govern the prevention of food poisoning without reference to the organisms known to be causal agents (and considered in Table 16); but information will be more comprehensive if preventive measures are related at least to the main groups of organisms and their characteristics.

The control of temperature during manufacture, storage, preparation and service in the factory, canteen and home is essential to keep bacterial numbers low. Suggested temperatures for the storage of various foods are given in Fig. 57.

Appendix A gives suggested outlines for lectures to various groups of people; e.g. Schedule 1 is intended for domestic audiences, Schedule 2 for non-technical professional food handlers. Appendix B is intended to help travellers with their choice of food, so that they remain free from gastroenteritis.

Appendix A

The following notes and headings for talks on food hygiene have been useful for various groups studying the safety and keeping quality of foodstuffs.

Schedule 1 may be used for one or two lectures with demonstrations and pictorial charts of outbreaks of food poisoning. Schedule 2 includes a course of ten talks with suggestions for charts, compiled by the late Miss I. J. Martin and Miss C. F. Scott.

SCHEDULE 1

Introduction

The term food poisoning describes a state in which the victim suffers an acute attack of abdominal pain and diarrhoea sometimes accompanied by vomiting and lasting usually 1–2 days, but sometimes a week or more. The onset is usually sudden and may start as early as 2 hours and up to 40 or more hours after eating the contaminated food.

Safe food will not cause food poisoning. Food may be harmful because it has taken up toxic metals such as zinc, copper or antimony; it may be poisonous itself, for example some fish, plants and fungi or it may induce allergic manifestations, but most food poisoning is caused by minute living organisms. These microorganisms are invisible except when viewed through a microscope. Their presence in food may be demonstrated either by food poisoning symptoms when the food looks, smells and tastes normal, or by spoilage when it looks, tastes and smells bad. At least five different groups of bacteria are concerned in food poisoning, and the symptoms and incubation periods vary from group to group. In general, the organisms must grow in the food to produce sufficient numbers to invade the body (infection) or to produce toxic substances either in the foodstuff or within the intestine. However, food may act as a vehicle for small numbers of bacterial agents causing more serious infections such as dysentery, typhoid and paratyphoid fevers or even for viral agents such as those causing infectious hepatitis and poliomyelitis.

Sources of food poisoning bacteria

1. Foods or food ingredients both imported and home-produced, as purchased or brought into the kitchen such as raw meat and poultry, rice and other cereals, other dehydrated food and seafoods.
2. Food handlers concerned with the manufacture and retail sale of food, those in catering and domestic kitchens: nose, throat and skin carriers of staphylococci and faecal excreters of salmonella and shigella organisms.
3. Food animals, poultry, pigs and other living creatures which infect the foods arising from them and intended both for human and for animal consumption. Domestic pets, vermin and flies which may be symptomless excreters in the environment of food preparation.
4. The factory, shop and kitchen which can harbour bacteria from all sources in benches, tables, cloths, boards, slicers, can openers and other equipment. Such contamination may be picked up by foods during preparation and after cooking.

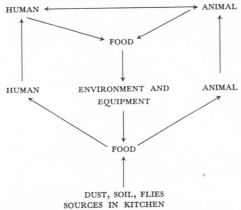

CHART—**Cycle of infection and contamination**

Food handlers and other living things

Foodstuffs, e.g. meat, poultry and seafoods

Surfaces and equipment

Bacterial agents of food poisoning

SALMONELLAE enter the kitchen on foods which are of animal origin such as meats, poultry and raw egg products, as well as from human excreters. Fertilizers and pet meats, which may be handled in the kitchen, are also sources of salmonellae. They are the commonest food-poisoning agents and the most serious. There is a 12 to 36 hour incubation period, the symptoms resemble gastric 'flu, and the illness lasts for 1 to 7 days.

STAPHYLOCOCCI come mainly from human carriers. The nose, throat, hand or skin lesion may harbour staphylococci able to cause food poisoning if the organisms are allowed to grow in foodstuffs, particularly those handled after cooking. While growing some staphylococci produce a toxin; the amount of toxin present will be proportional to the amount of bacterial growth, which depends on the length of time and the temperature at which the food has been stored. Staphylococci are frequently present in the milk of cows and goats; if the milk is not pasteurized the organisms may develop and produce toxin in the milk and it can be carried over into cream and cheese. Staphylococcal food poisoning has a 2 to 6 hour incubation period, the symptoms resemble acute sea-sickness and the illness lasts for 1 to 2 days.

CLOSTRIDIUM WELCHII produces hardy structures called spores which survive for a long time in dust, soil and excreta from both human and animals sources. The surfaces of raw meat and poultry are frequently contaminated with *Cl. welchii*. Some spores remain alive after boiling and other methods of cooking and grow readily in the cooked meat when it is cooled slowly and stored in a warm place. *Cl. welchii* will not grow in the presence of air; thus freshly cooked food is more able to support its growth, for the oxygen has been driven off during cooking. Furthermore, the spores may require heat to initiate germination and this is provided by cooking. Rolled joints are particularly dangerous because the spores are folded inside where conditions are suitable for anaerobic growth and the penetration of heat may be poor. The disease has an 8 to 22 hours incubation period, and the characteristic symptoms are abdominal pain and diarrhoea lasting 1 to 2 days. Toxin is produced in the intestine.

CLOSTRIDIUM BOTULINUM poisoning is rare in the United Kingdom. The spores are very heat resistant and the organism grows only in the absence of air. The contamination of canned and bottled foods, uncured and smoked fish (stored unfrozen), and preserved vegetables imperfectly prepared have given rise to outbreaks in the past. Incidents are reported from other countries. BACILLUS CEREUS is commonly found in foodstuffs and in the environment; it produces spores which can survive cooking and grow out in slowly cooling food particularly cereal products such as cornflour and rice. Toxin is formed in the food in proportion to the growth of the organism. The incubation period may be 2–4 hours up to 15 hours and the main symptom is vomiting.

VIBRIO PARAHAEMOLYTICUS occurs in warm coastal waters and various sea foods and it may pass from raw to cooked foods. It is a common cause of food poisoning in Japan and is reported from other countries also. The incubation period is approximately 15 hours and the illness includes profuse diarrhoea and vomiting which may last five or more days.

Other organisms, such as certain streptococci, *Proteus* and those in the Providence group are sometimes suspected to cause food poisoning when reaching abnormal numbers in food.

ESCHERICHIA COLI is known to cause diarrhoea in adults as well as in infants and the number of types found to be enteropathogenic is increasing.

Prevention

(a) Education and care of food handlers.
(b) Animal care.
(c) Vigilance: (i) imported food, (ii) home-produced food: farming, slaughtering, manufacture, catering.
(d) Care of equipment and cleanliness.

Conditions

Micro-organisms causing food poisoning must be able to grow in the food, which is known as the vehicle of infection; the prevention of growth is an important control measure. Bacteria increase by doubling in number every 10 to 30 minutes in ideal conditions. Most bacteria will grow at varying rates within the temperature range of 5 °C (41 °F) to 50 °C (122 °F). The most favourable temperature is about 37 °C (98·6 °F)—the temperature of the human body. Much of the food eaten by man is favourable for growth, for example, meat and meat products, poultry, eggs and egg products, milk and milk products.

Factors which encourage growth are high moisture, low salt (although staphylococci can tolerate more salt than other pathogenic bacteria) low acid, low fat and moderate sugar. Growth is repressed by heat, cold and dehydration, and by high concentrations of salt, sugar, acid and fat.

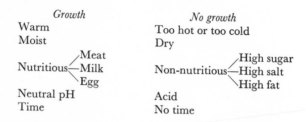

Growth	No growth
Warm	Too hot or too cold
Moist	Dry
Nutritious—Meat/Milk/Egg	Non-nutritious—High sugar/High salt/High fat
Neutral pH	Acid
Time	No time

Foods which do and do not encourage bacterial growth

The type of food is significant because some organisms will live and multiply readily in one type of food and others in another. For example, staphylococci grow in high salt concentrations, whereas salmonellae and *Cl. welchii* do not; thus staphylococcal food poisoning is frequently caused by semi-preserved salted meats. *Cl. welchii* grows rapidly in boiled fresh meat which is cooled slowly. Certain foods will not allow growth of food-poisoning organisms, for example those which are acid such as sauces, pickles and some soft drinks. Foods with a high sugar content, jams, syrups and honey, and foods with a high fat content discourage growth of bacteria, although they may survive. In dried or frozen foods organisms cannot multiply but a proportion of those already present before freezing or dehydration will survive.

Measures to control bacterial growth

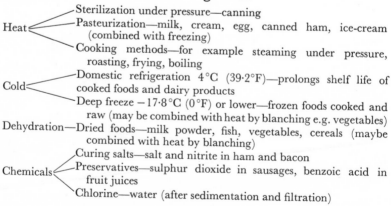

Heat
— Sterilization under pressure—canning
— Pasteurization—milk, cream, egg, canned ham, ice-cream (combined with freezing)
— Cooking methods—for example steaming under pressure, roasting, frying, boiling

Cold
— Domestic refrigeration 4 °C (39·2 °F)—prolongs shelf life of cooked foods and dairy products
— Deep freeze −17·8 °C (0 °F) or lower—frozen foods cooked and raw (may be combined with heat by blanching e.g. vegetables)

Dehydration—Dried foods—milk powder, fish, vegetables, cereals (maybe combined with heat by blanching)

Chemicals
— Curing salts—salt and nitrite in ham and bacon
— Preservatives—sulphur dioxide in sausages, benzoic acid in fruit juices
— Chlorine—water (after sedimentation and filtration)

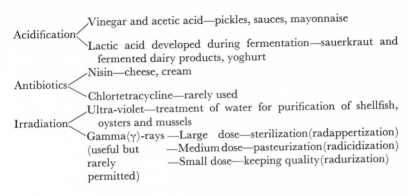

Acidification— Vinegar and acetic acid—pickles, sauces, mayonnaise
Lactic acid developed during fermentation—sauerkraut and fermented dairy products, yoghurt

Antibiotics— Nisin—cheese, cream
Chlortetracycline—rarely used

Irradiation— Ultra-violet—treatment of water for purification of shellfish, oysters and mussels
Gamma(γ)-rays —Large dose—sterilization(radappertization)
(useful but —Medium dose—pasteurization(radicidization)
rarely —Small dose—keeping quality(radurization)
permitted)

Thus milk is made safe by pasteurization, ultra heat treatment or sterilization, ice-cream by pasteurization, quick cooling and freezing, bulked egg by pasteurization and water by filtration and chlorination.

The Hygiene of food including purchase and preparation

PURCHASING AND SHOPS. More food should not be purchased than the amount which can be stored in the available deep freeze cabinet or domestic refrigerator (4 °C, 39·2 °F).

STORAGE. Deep freeze storage keeps food safe for many months and even years, but domestic refrigeration can keep food palatable for a limited number of days only.

SHOPS. The shop or supermarket should have chill cabinets (4 °C, 39·2 °F) for susceptible foods such as cold cooked meats and raw meat or poultry; the raw products should be well separated from cooked meatstuffs.

SLICED MEATS. Susceptible foods such as semi-preserved cooked meats and pies should not be handled nor shown in the shop window; sliced and weighed quantities prepared under specially hygienic conditions should be wrapped in cellophane and kept chilled before sale. In fact there should be no opportunity of cross-contamination between raw and cooked materials.

SAUSAGES. Sausages should not be on sale alongside cooked products, and they should be kept cold.

FISH. Fish should be bought from enclosed shops with chilled cabinets or chilled window displays.

CANS. Canned goods should be in good condition; when the containers are rusted or damaged they should not be on sale. It must be emphasized that large cans of ham and similar products which are not sterile should be refrigerated; the canner's instruction to 'keep cold' implies that the pack is perishable.

CREAM CAKES. Imitation cream cakes should be kept under chilled storage for a limited period of sale (1 day). Fresh cream should be chilled unless long storage is assured by in-bottle pasteurization. There should be ample cold and cool storage space both for raw and cooked products in the kitchen.

The food handler

PERSONAL HYGIENE. The nose, mouth and skin can be sources of staphylococci which produce toxin in foods; thus cooked foods able to support growth should not be touched by hand. Salmonellae, dysentery bacilli and *Clostridium welchii* may be excreted in stools so hands should be washed after using the WC.

HANDS. Hands should be washed well after, as well as before, handling foods because food-poisoning organisms can be picked up from many raw foodstuffs and transferred to cooked and other foods. Hands should be dried on paper towels or the continuous roller towel. Lesions must be covered and persons with septic lesions should not handle food.

HABITS. Habits should be good, no smoking while handling food, no tasting of food by sampling with the fingers; spoons used for tasting should be immediately washed in hot water.

HANDKERCHIEFS. Paper handkerchiefs should be available and after use disposed of in a box or cellophane bag kept in a convenient place.

NAILS AND CLOTHES. Nails should be short and clean and clothing clean; personal clothes should not be washed in the kitchen.

NO-TOUCH TECHNIQUES. There should be little or no actual man-handling of susceptible foods, particularly after recent lesions on the hands.

SOAPS AND HAND CREAMS. Bactericidal soaps and hand creams are useful, because the hands must be kept in good condition. Cracks, blemishes and broken nails will all harbour bacteria, and good hand cream containing a bactericidal substance should be used after washing.

TOILET FACILITIES. Pedal-operated flushes and taps, and easily cleaned metal fittings should be used wherever possible.

Environment of the kitchen

LAYOUT. Work benches, cooking and hand-washing facilities as well as the sink unit should be conveniently placed and well lit. So far as possible there should be separate work areas for raw and cooked food; for large scale catering this is essential and should include separate equipment and personnel in the different areas.

SURFACES. Smooth and impermeable surfaces are easy to clean and thus the number of bacteria in the environment will be reduced; stainless steel and Formica, even good enamel are preferable to all other types of material. Boards should be made from one piece of hardwood for ease of cleaning and disinfection; Formica, rubber or other materials should be used in place of wood for cutting boards.

HOT WATER. There should be a plentiful supply of hot water.

STORAGE. A cold room or refrigeration and deep freeze facilities are required, also a well-ventilated, cool cupboard or larder. There should be provision for the rapid cooling of bulks of meat, poultry and other foods to be refrigerated, such as a special chill room with extraction fans or a fan in the larder. An internal cupboard may be used for canned and bottled foods. There should be ample space for cleaning materials and also for storing vegetables, preferably outside the main kitchen, in a cool place away from direct sunlight. Food required to be served hot should be maintained at a temperature above 65 °C.

EQUIPMENT. Equipment should be bought with a view to easy cleaning, and sited for ease of cleaning and accessibility; it should be easily taken apart and reassembled and maintained in good repair.

CLEANING EQUIPMENT. All parts should be freed from food debris (if necessary using a brush) with hot soapy or detergent water and rinsed with very hot water. Hypochlorites and other suitable chemical agents, or steam, may be used; adequate time for contact should be allowed.

NAIL BRUSHES. Nail brushes should not be harsh; nylon and plastic are recommended so that they can be disinfected.

PAPER. The use of disposable paper instead of cloths for mopping up is important to prevent spreading contamination from place to place by a moist much-handled cloth.

WASHING-UP. There should be three stages; pre-cleaning, a good cleaning detergent, and a really hot water rinse; where it is impossible to obtain hot water a bactericidal detergent should be considered, or a final rinse in hypochlorite solution.

GARBAGE. Garbage can be discarded by burning in the boiler or by wrapping and placing in pedal-operated bins or dustbins; cans should be washed free from remains of food. Garbage receptacles should be kept dry and clean; when they are damp bacteria can multiply in the waste, thus creating spoilage smells. They should be covered and in the shade.

Paper sacks are useful and popular, also the waste disposal system attached to the sink, although there are limitations to its use, as cans and clothing materials cannot be disposed of in this way.

FLIES. Flies should be denied access to dustbins otherwise eggs will be laid and the grubs will hatch in suitable refuse; flies must be kept out of the kitchens also.

Cooking and preparation

POULTRY. Poultry may harbour food-poisoning organisms on the skin, in offal and inside the carcass. Thus care should be taken where and how birds are prepared, surfaces and utensils should be well cleaned after use, and the hands washed well after handling the raw materials. Cloths should not be used to wipe carcasses either inside or outside, or to cover poultry or meat. Frozen meat and poultry should be thawed properly before cooking. If foods are not to be eaten freshly cooked and hot they must be cooled quickly and refrigerated.

PET MEAT. Pet meat, raw or in open packs, frequently contains food-poisoning organisms; it should not be handled, but utensils should be kept for that purpose only and boiled after use.

SAUSAGES. Sausages, raw scraps and minced meat may be contaminated with salmonellae. Great care should be taken when preparing sausages for cooking. If they are pricked (now said to be unnecessary) the fork should be washed immediately with very hot water. Sausages should be well cooked.

EGG POWDERS. Dried products such as meringue powder and powdered egg should be handled with care and used only for well-cooked products. Prepared cake mixes should not include egg products such as egg white or whole egg powder.

SHELL EGGS. Duck's eggs should not be used unless cooked thoroughly and all receptacles and utensils scalded after use.

MEAT PIES. Casseroles, cottage and shepherd's pies, steak and kidney puddings and pies, pasties and similar dishes should be prepared freshly from raw meat. If there is likely to be any delay in using cooked meat for pies, steaming under pressure is the best way to ensure the destruction of heat-resistant organisms; it is a safe method of cooking. If left-overs are used 'warmed-up' they must be cooked thoroughly to boiling point to destroy contaminants and toxins which may have been formed. All cooked meats should be hurried from cooker to refrigerator and back again.

ROLLED MEATS. Rolled joints are particularly prone to give rise to *Cl. welchii* food poisoning, because spores on the outer surfaces are rolled inside where they are more likely to survive. Such joints should be cooked thoroughly and eaten freshly cooked; they ought not to be allowed to cool slowly and stored at atmospheric temperature.

COLD COOKED MEATS. A very large proportion of food poisoning is caused by cold cooked meats; great care should be taken with their handling and storage.

TONGUE AND HAM. These products and particularly tongue, are subject to contamination by hand after cooking; the skinning of tongues while warm followed by long storage at atmospheric temperature encourages contamination and bacterial multiplication. Tongues should be heated again after skinning and pressing.

SALADS AND FRUITS. Salad vegetables including watercress and lettuce, and dessert fruits which cannot be peeled, should be well washed, preferably in water containing hypochlorite.

SANDWICHES. Sandwiches should be made as near the time required as possible; if prepared the night before they should be refrigerated in a container overnight.

COOKED RICE. Cooked rice should not be stored overnight unless refrigerated. Care must be taken with bulks of rice required in eating places specializing in curries and other dishes both for sitdown and take-away meals.

SEAFOODS. Oysters, mussels and other shellfish should be obtained only from reputable sources. After thawing, frozen cooked prawns and shrimps should be stored cold until required. Care is needed to prevent cross-contamination from raw to cooked food.

SUMMER. If the weather is hot all precautions should be strengthened and the foodstuffs which are prone to give rise to food poisoning should be excluded from the menu.

Points to remember

1. All cold cooked meats to be refrigerated and not handled.
2. Raw foods, such as meats and poultry to be thawed properly, cooked well and eaten hot or cooled quickly and refrigerated.
3. All equipment to be cleaned well and disinfected preferably by heat.

SCHEDULE 2

Food-borne disease is caused by the consumption of contaminated food or drink (see 'Types of food poisoning' below). Food which smells good, looks good and tastes good can still cause food poisoning.*

Types of food poisoning (SESSION 1)

1. Food itself may be poisonous; for example, some plants, fungi and shell-fish.
2. Allergic or sensitivity reactions to certain foods.
3. Micro-organisms, most commonly bacteria, or the poisons they form (called toxins) present in food or drink, some of which survive the heat of cooking.
4. Chemical contamination may occur during food preparation. Acid foods can dissolve metal from containers or utensils; for example, apples left in a galvanized container can cause zinc poisoning.
5. Parasites in animals which may be present in meat; for example, trichinella.

Types 1, 2, 4 and 5 occur occasionally, but the third is the commonest cause and can be prevented by care in the production and handling of food.

Bacteria

These organisms are minute living cells, varying in shape and visible only through a microscope. They are present everywhere. Most bacteria are harmless and even useful to man, but a small proportion are dangerous.

Given the right conditions, bacteria will divide into two every 20 to 30 minutes, so that one organism can develop into many millions within 12 hours.

Characteristics of illness

The symptoms are diarrhoea and abdominal pain, usually but not always accompanied by vomiting, coming on within 2 to 36 hours of eating food.

* *Note:* Information on yearly incidence of food poisoning may be obtained from the area health officer.

CHART—**Causes of food poisoning**

1. Foods   Plants, fungi, some shell-fish
2. Allergies
3. Micro-organisms

BACTERIA	
Small dose*	Dysentery bacilli
(spread readily)	
Large dose**	Salmonella
(usually after growth in food)	Staphylococcus
	Cl. welchii
	Cl. botulinum
	B. cereus
	V. parahaemolyticus

VIRUSES
Small dose*

4. Chemicals

Zinc
Copper
Tin
Alkaloids
Pesticides

5. Parasites

Trichinella
Taenia

* Small dose = few organisms only.
** Large dose = thousands to millions of organisms.

Conditions which affect the growth of bacteria (SESSION 2)

1. *Food:* Much of the protein food eaten by man is favourable for the growth of bacteria; for example, meat and meat products, poultry, eggs, milk and milk products.

2. *Temperature:* Many bacteria will grow at varying rates within the temperature range of 5 to 50 °C (41 to 122 °F). The most favourable temperature for food-poisoning bacteria is 37 °C (98·6 °F), the temperature of the human body; spoilage bacteria grow at lower . temperatures.

3. *Time:* When food and temperature provide favourable conditions for bacterial growth, time is needed for multiplication to take place.

4. *Moisture:* Moisture is necessary for growth, but most bacteria can survive indefinitely when dry, as in powdered food.

5. *Atmosphere:* Most bacteria require air to grow actively but some can multiply only in the absence of oxygen.

The danger zone

Optimum temperatures for bacterial growth are 20 to 45 °C (68 to 113 °F). Outside these temperature limits the bacteria which infect man and animals grow slowly.

The safety zone

Extreme cold will not kill all bacteria, but most will cease to multiply under refrigerated storage and none will grow in the freezer.

Effect of heat

Bacteria are destroyed by temperatures above 63 °C (145·4 °F) if held for sufficient length of time in cooking processes, due to irreversible protein changes (coagulation of whole egg), and in the pasteurization of milk; spores may not be killed by these treatments.

Toxins

Poisonous substances are produced in food by some bacteria, such as staphylococci, *B. cereus* and *Cl. botulinum.* They may be destroyed readily by heat (toxins of *Cl. botulinum*) or they may not be destroyed completely unless boiled for about 30 minutes (staphylococcal enterotoxin).

Spores

Hardy structures are produced by bacteria such as *Cl. welchii, Cl. botulinum* and *B. cereus.* They are not killed by temperatures which kill bacteria; some spores survive boiling. They remain dormant in dust and soil for long periods.

Food-poisoning bacteria (SESSION 3)

There are seven main types of bacteria causing food poisoning today.

1. *Salmonella*	infection by living bacteria in food.
2. *Staphylococcus*	toxin from growth of bacteria in food.
3. *Cl. welchii*	toxin released in intestine from living bacteria swallowed in food.
4. *Cl. botulinum*	toxin from growth of bacteria in food.
5. *B. cereus*	toxin from growth of bacteria in food.
6. *V. parahaemolyticus*	infection by living bacteria in food.
7. *Esch. coli*	infection by living bacteria in food.

Salmonella

This is the commonest cause of food poisoning and the most serious.

Source: Carried in the human and animal intestine, and excreted in stools. Likely to come into the kitchen on raw foods of animal origin; for example, meat, poultry, pet meat, sausages, egg products or to be brought in by human and animal excreta and fertilizers. Insects, birds, vermin and domestic pets may play a part.

Cause of illness: The living bacteria in food.

Illness: Begins 12 to 36 hours after eating contaminated food. Symptoms include fever, headache, abdominal pains, diarrhoea and vomiting. The illness lasts from 1 to 7 or 8 days and can be fatal in the elderly, very young or sick people.

Kitchen control:

1. Kitchen hygiene
   (a) Separation of raw from cooked foods, particularly meat and poultry, using different surfaces and equipment to prevent cross-contamination by boards, cutting and mincing machines, cloths and kitchen tools.
   (b) Thorough cleaning of all surfaces, equipment and tools.
2. Care of personal hygiene by washing hands before and after handling food—especially raw meat and poultry.
3. Cold storage of food to prevent multiplication of bacteria.

Staphylococcus

Staphylococci are a common cause of food poisoning.

Source: Comes mainly from the skin of human carriers and can be found in the nose, on the hands, in the throat, in boils, carbuncles, whitlows, styes, septic lesions, burns and scratches. Also comes from the raw milk of cows and goats; the organisms and toxin can be carried over to cream and cheese made from raw milk.

Cause of illness: A toxin produced by the bacteria as they grow in food.

Illness: Begins 2 to 6 hours after eating contaminated food. Symptoms include acute vomiting, pain in abdomen, diarrhoea and sometimes collapse; there is no fever. The illness lasts not more than 24 hours, and is seldom fatal.

Kitchen control:

1. Care of personal hygiene; it is impossible to sterilize the hands, therefore cooked food should not be touched by the hands.
2. Cold storage of food to prevent multiplication of bacteria.

3. Kitchen hygiene to prevent bacteria becoming numerous in equipment, boards, cutting and mincing machines, cloths, Savoy bags and other tools; clean thoroughly after use.

Clostridium welchii

Clostridium welchii is also a common cause of food poisoning.

Source: Found in the human and animal intestine, soil, dust and flies. Raw meat and poultry and some dried products are frequently contaminated with *Cl. welchii*; the spores can survive normal cooking temperatures. The organism grows without oxygen.

Cause of illness: Large numbers of bacilli growing in food. The spores remain active after boiling and slow roasting, and grow readily in cooked meat cooled slowly or stored in a warm place. Large numbers of bacilli build up quickly under these conditions. A toxin is released in the intestine.

Illness: Begins 8 to 22 hours after eating contaminated food. Symptoms include abdominal pain and diarrhoea, but rarely vomiting. The illness lasts from 1 to 2 days; it may be fatal in elderly and sick people.

Kitchen control:

1. Consideration of cooking methods and size of joints.
2. Rapid cooling to prevent multiplication of bacteria.
3. Cold storage of food to prevent multiplication of bacteria.
4. Separation of raw from cooked food to prevent cross-contamination.
5. Kitchen hygiene; thorough cleaning of all surfaces and equipment, boards, cutting machines, cloths and other tools after use. Regular removal of soil from vegetable store and preparation area and dust from cereals in dry goods store.

Clostridium botulinum

Clostridium botulinum is an uncommon cause of food poisoning.

Source: Found in soil, meat and fish in some areas; the spores survive cooking and other processes. The organism grows without oxygen.

Cause of illness: A toxin produced by the bacilli as they grow in food.

Illness: Begins 24 to 72 hours after eating contaminated food. There is fatigue, headache and dizziness. There may be diarrhoea at first but not later. The nervous system is attacked and vision and speech are disturbed. Death often occurs within 8 days, unless antitoxin is given soon after onset of illness.

Kitchen control:
1. Avoid home preservation of meat, poultry, game and fish except by freezing.
2. Avoid eating raw and fermented fish.
3. Discourage smoking and curing of fish in certain areas of the world where the organism is common.
4. Careful inspection of cans and contents.
5. Care with curing solutions.

Bacillus cereus

Bacillus cereus may be a common cause of food poisoning.
Source: Found in soil, dust, cereals, vegetables, dairy products and many other foods; the spores survive cooking. The organism grows best with oxygen.
Cause of illness: A toxin produced by the bacilli as they grow in food.
Illness: Begins 2 to 3 (or even up to 15) hours after eating contaminated food. There is vomiting and sometimes diarrhoea later. The illness lasts 1 to 2 days or less.
Kitchen control:
1. Avoid storage of cooked bulks of rice and other cereals.
2. Rapid cooling to prevent multiplication of bacilli.
3. Cold storage of food to prevent multiplication.
4. Kitchen hygiene; the thorough cleaning of all surfaces, equipment and tools. Regular removal of cereal dust from storage and preparation areas.

Vibrio parahaemolyticus

Vibrio parahaemolyticus is a common cause of food poisoning in Japan; occasionally reported from other countries.
Source: Found in sea creatures and coastal waters.
Cause of illness: The living bacteria in raw and cooked seafoods such as fish, prawns, crabs and other shell-fish.
Illness: Begins approximately 15 hours after eating contaminated food. Symptoms include acute diarrhoea, abdominal pain and vomiting with fever. The illness lasts for 2 to 5 days or more.
Kitchen control:
1. Care that cooking methods destroy the organisms.
2. Separation of raw and cooked food to prevent cross-contamination from raw to cooked products by hands and other methods.
3. Rapid cooling to prevent multiplication of vibrios.
4. Cold storage of food to prevent multiplication.

5. Kitchen hygiene; thorough cleaning of all surfaces, equipment and tools after use.

Escherichia coli

   Escherichia coli may be a common cause of food poisoning (also thought to be associated with traveller's diarrhoea).

Source: Carried in the human and animal intestine and excreted in stools. Likely to come into the kitchen in the human and animal excreter and in raw foods of animal origin; for example, meat, poultry and pet meat. The part played by insects, birds, vermin and domestic pets is not yet known.

Cause of illness: The living bacteria in food.

Illness: Begins 18 to 48 hours after eating contaminated food (or drinking polluted water). Symptoms include pain and diarrhoea and sometimes pyrexia and vomiting. The illness lasts from 1 to 5 days.

Kitchen control:

1. Care of personal hygiene by washing hands before and after handling food—especially raw meat and poultry.
2. Care of water used for washing salad and vegetables.
3. Separation of raw from cooked food to prevent cross-contamination.
4. Kitchen hygiene; thorough cleaning of all surfaces, equipment and tools after use.

How bacteria reach food—contamination (Session 4)

Foods which encourage growth of bacteria

   Raw and cooked meat and poultry, foods with meat as a base, soups, stocks, gravies, 'made-up' meat dishes; also eggs, milk and milk products, fresh and imitation cream.

Foods and liquids which are safe

   Water—filtered, chlorinated and bottled mineral waters.

   Milk—pasteurized, ultra heat treated or sterilized.

   Ice-cream—mix pasteurized, cooled rapidly and kept cold until frozen: manufacture controlled by regulations.

   Whole egg mix in bulk—pasteurized.

   Most canned foods (large cans of ham are not sterile and must be kept cold), bread, flour, jams and honey, pickles and acid fruits, fats.

How bacteria reach food

Raw foodstuffs: The organisms can be carried in the animal intestine and may be spread on to the carcass. Therefore meat and poultry can come into the kitchen already contaminated with salmonellae and clostridia. Contact between carcasses and between meats will spread bacteria, and food handlers may pick up food-poisoning organisms from the foods they handle.

Food handlers: Careless handling during transport, manufacture, preparation and service may add and spread bacteria to food. Hands can transfer food-poisoning germs from raw to cooked foods. Personal bacteria from the nose, mouth, skin, stool and hands can contaminate food.

Environment:

1. Unclean kitchen surfaces and equipment can harbour bacteria and so contaminate other foods; bacteria from raw meat and poultry can be passed to the cooked foods.
2. Flies, rats, mice, cats, dogs, birds and other animals and pets can carry bacteria to food.
3. Dust and soil with dried organisms or excreta can contaminate food.

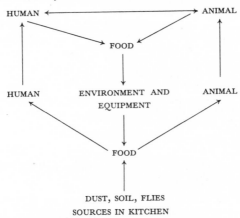

CHART—**Cycle of infection and contamination**

DUST, SOIL, FLIES
SOURCES IN KITCHEN
Food handlers and other living things
Foodstuffs, e.g., meat, poultry and seafoods
Surfaces and equipment

CHART—Prevention of food poisoning

1. Prevent spread of contamination in the kitchen.
   (a) Separation of raw and cooked food to avoid cross-contamination.
   (b) Care on part of food handler.
   (c) Cleanliness of kitchen environment.
2. Prevent bacteria already in food from growing and spreading.
   (a) Cold storage facilities must be adequate and efficiently maintained.
   (b) Avoid long storage in warmth—close time gaps between preparation and serving.
   (c) Provide facilities for rapid cooling.

   } In the retail store and in the kitchen.

3. Cook to destroy most bacteria (but not spores), with particular attention to:
   (a) Careful preparation and adequate cooking.
   If possible, serve at once. If not:
   (b) Keep hot; or
   (c) Cool rapidly and store cold.
   (d) Avoid recontamination.

Personal hygiene (SESSION 5)

It is the food handler's responsibility to take scrupulous care that personal bacteria are not added to food. Bacteria from the following sources can be passed to food by the hands:

1. Secretions from the nose, throat and skin, dust and dandruff from the hair.
2. Excreta from the bowel.
3. Other people's secretions and excreta.
4. Liquor from raw meat and poultry and from other foods, including powdered foods.
5. Utensils and equipment.
6. Cloths—tea towels, dishcloths, meat cloths.

Personal hygiene can break the chain of infection in the following ways:

Hands

Hands should be kept in good condition, free from roughness.
1. *Washing:* Thorough washing with hot water and soap is essential after using the WC, immediately before, during and after food preparation, after handling raw meat or poultry and after

using a handkerchief. Hand washing should not be done in kitchen sinks. Wash-basins should be:

(a) In or adjacent to a toilet

(b) In the kitchen preparation area

they should be supplied with hot and cold water, a soap dispenser, nail brush and an individual method of hand drying. Hand cream with added disinfectant should be available.

Hands are NOT sterile after washing.

2. *Nails:* keep short and very clean.

3. *Cuts and abrasions:* cover with a non-porous dressing or Newskin and a fingerstall or glove if necessary. Persons with septic lesions should not work with food until the infection is completely healed.

4. *Fingers:* do not lick when tasting or serving food or separating sheets of paper.

Good habits

Take care not to touch the nose, hair or face; avoid sneezing and coughing near food; maintain a high standard of bodily cleanliness.

Smoking

Smoking must be prohibited in premises where there is uncovered food.

Handkerchiefs

Handkerchiefs carry infection from nasal secretions. They can contaminate hands and clothing and, indirectly, foods. Paper tissues are useful and easily disposable.

Hair

Hair should be well covered with cloth, net or paper caps.

Clothing

Clean overalls and aprons are essential; changed regularly and frequently.

Health

Illness, particularly diarrhoea, vomiting, throat and skin infections, should be reported. Severe septic conditions should also be reported.

Purchasing and storage (SESSION 6)

Purchasing

The standards of hygiene maintained by the supplier should be noted, such as cold and chilled storage, separation of raw and cooked foods, handling of unwrapped raw and cooked foods, cleanliness of premises and equipment and type of equipment.

Perishable foods

Raw and cooked meat and poultry, milk, cream and fish should be bought in quantities sufficient for one day only unless there is ample refrigerated space. Meat and fish should not be refrigerated for more than three days.

Non-perishable foods

Dry goods, preserves, canned foods should be bought in reasonable quantities. Avoid overstocking; there is danger from vermin and deterioration where storage facilities are poor. These products should be stored in a dry, well ventilated storeroom.

Storage of perishable foods

The following foods must be refrigerated: raw and cooked meat and poultry, dairy products, fats, fish, jellies and trifles.

Raw meat and poultry must be refrigerated on delivery. Store raw and cooked meat and poultry separately to prevent cross-contamination.

Refrigerator

The temperature should be 1 to 4 °C (33·8 to 39·2 °F), checked with a thermometer. Bacteria are not destroyed but those that are significant to man do not grow readily.
1. Packing
    (a) Do not overcrowd the shelves and prevent circulation of cold air.
    (b) Use the coldest part for the most susceptible foods.
    (c) Cover food to prevent loss of moisture and transfer of smells.
    (d) Ensure that all containers are dry and clean; milk bottles should be wiped.
2. Food must be cooled before refrigeration, otherwise the humidity and temperature will rise in the refrigerator.

3. Open the door as little as possible and close it quickly.
4. Defrost and clean weekly.
5. Regular servicing is essential.

Storage of non-perishable food—storeroom and larder
1. Keep cool, well ventilated and dry.
2. Proof against vermin and flies.
3. Surfaces of shelves, walls and floors should be easy to clean.
4. Arrange packs in an orderly manner:
    (a) Food 18 inches (450 mm) from floor unless in mobile metal bins.
    (b) Stock rotated—dated on delivery.

Deep freeze unit
The temperature, $-18\,°C(-0·4\,°F)$, is much lower than the refrigerator. Use for long-term storage; food must be well protected. Defrost periodically; regular servicing is essential.

Read and follow instruction on packs of frozen foods. Thawed food should not be refrozen.

Vegetables
Keep in cool storage, preferably screened from the kitchen to keep soil bacteria away from food preparation and cooking areas.

Rapid cooling larders
Rooms with extractor fans and adequate intake of air through filter pads to give moving air currents should be available. Impervious materials should be used for all surfaces.

Food preparation—cooking and serving (SESSION 7)

Remember
1. Conditions which favour growth of bacteria must be avoided, especially the length of time food is left at temperatures suitable for bacterial growth.
2. Foods which are sources of food-poisoning bacteria and those which encourage growth need special care; for example, raw and cooked meat, foods with meat as a base, made-up meat and fish dishes, sandwiches, raw and cooked poultry, sweets with lightly cooked or raw egg, milk products, and fresh and imitation cream. Keep pet foods out of commercial kitchens; in the home,

store apart from household foods and use separate utensils.
Cook well.
3. Particular care is needed in the summer months (June to
October); bacteria grow readily in warm weather.

Kitchen practice

Personal hygiene

Bacteria from all sources can be passed to food by hands. Wash
frequently before and during food preparation. In spite of washing,
do not handle cooked foods.

Cooking techniques

Heat penetrates slowly and is lost slowly in traditional cooking
methods; with microwaves heat penetration is rapid but not
necessarily uniform. Infra-red rays are used for browning only.
Cooking does not always destroy bacterial spores or even bacteria,
particularly in rolled and stuffed joints, poultry, large meat pies
and sausages.
1. Avoid partial cooking.
2. Cool cooked food rapidly and refrigerate within 1½ hours.
Cooling can be speeded up by:
  (a) Provision of rapid cooling larders.
  (b) Breaking up bulk and placing in shallow containers in a
     moving current of air.
  (c) Limiting the size of joints to not more than 6 lb (2·7 kg).
3. Avoid reheating food. If it is essential the food must be boiled or
recooked thoroughly in all parts.
4. Keep hot food hot and serve quickly.
5. *Safe cooking methods*   *Less safe methods*
   Pressure cooking   Boiling
   Grilling   Stewing
   Frying   Braising
   Roasting of small or thin joints   Roasting of large bulky and
                                       rolled joints

Kitchen equipment

Ease of cleaning is an important factor in selecting all surfaces,
equipment and utensils.
1. Keep surfaces, equipment and utensils clean and in good
repair; they should not be old or worn.

CHART—**Food-borne infection in the kitchen and methods of control**

FOOD	*Hazard*	*Action in kitchen*
DELIVERY	Raw meat and poultry	Immediate cold storage Care in handling
PREPARATION	Hands	Wash thoroughly and frequently
	Surfaces, containers, equipment, kitchen tools, boards and cloths.	1. Clean thoroughly with hot water and detergent. 2. Heat and chemical disinfection; e.g. hypochlorite solutions (combined with detergent or after washing)
COOKING PROCESSES	*Less safe methods* Boiling Stewing Braising	*Safer methods* Pressure cooking Roasting Grilling Frying
	Large bulks of food	Divide into small quantities
COOLING AFTER COOKING	Long slow cooling	Rapid cooling within 1½ hours. Refrigerate
SERVING	Long storage in warmth	Serve freshly cooked. Keep hot
	Contamination from hands	Do not handle cooked food
	Contamination from equipment	Suitable equipment kept clean
COOKED MEAT		Serve hot and keep hot, above 63 °C (145·4 °F), or cool quickly, serve cold; keep cold, below 5 °C (41 °F),
	KEEP TIME SHORT 1. Between cooking and eating 2. Between cooking and cold storage 3. Between cold storage, serving and cold storage of remainder	

2. Slicing machines, mincing machines and can openers require frequent and thorough cleaning; they must be easy to dismantle and reassemble. In-plant cleaning may be necessary for fixed parts of equipment.
3. Use separate boards for raw meat, cooked meat and vegetables. Choose appropriate materials for ease of cleaning; for example, synthetic and/or natural rubber hardened with plastic fillers, high molecular weight, medium-density polyethylene or phenolic fibre laminates.

For cleaning use hot water and detergent combined with or followed by a disinfecting agent such as hypochlorite.

Avoid cloths; use disposable paper instead.

Serving
1. Avoid exposure of susceptible foods in warm atmosphere. Keep cold food cold, below 5 °C (41 °F).
2. Avoid warm storage of cooked food. Keep hot food hot, above 63 °C (145·4 °F).
3. Keep displayed food cold and under cover.
4. Minimize handling of cooked foods; use suitable kitchen tools.
5. Use new clean paper for wrapping and covering food.
6. Keep animals and insects out of the kitchen.

Washing-up (SESSION 8)

Efficient washing-up is necessary to clean and remove bacteria from all dining room and kitchen equipment. The essential provisions are:

1. Good layout of washing-up area.
2. Correct temperature of wash and rinse water.
3. A good detergent suited to the type of water.
4. Orderly methods of work in rinsing, stacking, racking and storage.

Preparation

The aim is to remove as much food waste as possible before washing.
1. Cutlery should be rinsed.
2. Tableware should be scraped and rinsed.
3. Tableware should be stacked according to kind for hand-washing or racked according to kind for machine washing. Cutlery should be racked with bowls and prongs uppermost.

Methods

Dish-washing machine: The large machines operate automatically and provide:

1. A pre-rinse to soften and remove food particles. When using small machines this process must be done by hand.
2. A detergent wash, temperature 60°C (140°F); an automatic dispenser can be fitted.
3. A rinse at a higher temperature 82 to 87°C (180 to 190°F). Remove clean dry ware from racks and store.

Two- or three-sink method: Suitable for domestic and large-scale use.

1. Rinse, scrape or wipe off, with paper, food particles.
2. Wash in hot water, 46 to 50°C (115 to 122°F) with measured detergent or detergent/disinfectant.
3. Rinse in racks in hot water, 77 to 82°C (170 to 180°F) (maintained). Both wash and rinse waters should be changed as soon as they become soiled or lose temperature.
4. Rack for drying before storage.

One-sink or bowl method: Inefficient since crockery and cutlery may still be contaminated with bacteria.

Drying

When the hot rinse is at the right temperature, dishes in racks will air-dry in 30 to 40 seconds.

Cloths

Dish cloths and tea towels harbour bacteria and require daily disinfection, preferably by heat. They can contaminate hands, equipment and cutlery.

Paper

Disposable paper should be used in place of dish cloths and tea towels.

Storage

Covered storage should be provided.

Waste disposal (SESSION 9)

In kitchen

Food scraps on floors and surfaces encourage bacterial growth and attract vermin.

Waste can be collected:
1. In pedal-operated bins which can be emptied regularly and washed out.
2. In paper or plastic bags on pedal-operated stands. Bags can be sealed and put into dustbins, incinerated or collected by the local council.

Outside kitchen

Provide sufficient waste bins or paper sacks to prevent over-spilling.

Bins with well-fitting lids should be placed in shade on a stand 250 to 300 mm (10 to 12 inches) high above a concrete area with drainage, which can be hosed down. Wet-strength paper or plastic bags with lids should be wall-mounted to give good ground clearance for hosing down.

Paper waste is usually kept separately.

Tins should be rinsed, both ends removed and beaten flat.

Bins (other than for pig food) should be kept as dry as possible by wrapping wet waste.

Waste disposal unit

The unit is attached to the sink waste pipe. The ground refuse passes into the waste pipe and drain.

Vermin and fly control

Rats, mice and insects

Rats, mice, flies, cockroaches and ants are the most common pests.

If premises do not provide food and shelter, infestation is unlikely.

For extermination, seek expert advice from the local authority.

Flies, including bluebottles

Feet and hairs spread bacteria acquired from excreta and other waste.

Control:

1. Do not provide a breeding ground such as uncovered refuse bins. Bins (other than for pig food) should be kept as dry as possible.
2. Destroy flies by spraying the refuse area in summer to prevent breeding.
3. Prevent access to kitchen and food by fly-proof windows, doors and ventilators. Cover food.

Cockroaches

Active at night. Attracted to warm places, such as heating pipes. Seal off crevices which provide hiding places.

Close-fitting lids prevent access to food.

Treat area with suitable insecticide.

Sprays and powders

Care must be taken to prevent pesticides reaching food, preparation surfaces and equipment.

Premises (SESSION 10)

The layout of a kitchen must be planned with the principles of hygiene in mind, with regard to the sources of food-poisoning bacteria (human, raw foods, environment) and also the importance of hot and cold storage.

Floors

Durable, non-slip surfaces should be impervious to moisture and easy to clean. Equipment preferably is raised or mobile to allow floor to be cleaned underneath.

Walls

Smooth, impervious walls should reduce condensation and be easy to clean. Junctions of wall and floor should be coved for easy cleaning and equipment fixed away from the wall to allow for cleaning.

Ceiling

The surface which encloses the inside of the roof should be smooth, anticondensation and easy to clean.

Lighting

Illumination must be good, both natural and artificial, particularly over work and preparation areas, sinks and cooking equipment. Shadows should be avoided.

Ventilation

Good natural and mechanical ventilation is necessary to prevent a rise in temperature and humidity.

Sanitary convenience

Toilets must not open directly into food-preparation rooms. Foot-operated flushes are desirable.

Wash-basins should be available:

1. In or adjacent to the toilet.
2. In kitchen preparation areas.

They should be supplied with:

(a) Hot and cold water; foot operation is preferable.
(b) Soap dispenser.
(c) Nail brush with plastic or Nylon back and bristle (wood harbours bacteria).
(d) An individual method of hand drying, such as paper towels, continuous roll towels or hot-air dryers. Roller towels (old type) should not be used because there is danger of cross-infection.
(e) Antiseptic hand cream should be available.

Cloakroom

Outer clothing must not be kept in the kitchen; adequate hanging space for the number of staff employed must be provided in a separate room.

Food preparation surfaces

Wood is unsuitable because it is too difficult to clean. The best materials are stainless steel or a laminate.

Chopping boards

Wood is still used but it constitutes a hazard. Compressed rubber is available, or plastic for light use. Thorough cleaning is necessary after use, followed by a disinfectant or 'sanitizing' agent, such as hypochlorite. Separate 'boards' are required for raw meat, cooked meat and vegetables.

Sinks

Stainless steel with sink and drainer in one piece is recommended. There should be separate sinks for vegetable preparation.

Refrigerator and/or cold room

Facilities for cold storage are essential for safety and they must be of adequate size. There should be adjustable metal shelves in the cold room.

Fixed equipment

The design must allow easy cleaning, and avoid ledges, nooks and crannies; fix away from walls.

Facilities

Rapid cooling is most essential.

Summary of preventive care

1. Do not touch with the hands:
cooked, prepared food—particularly meats and poultry.

2. Keep time short between:
cooking and eating
cooking and refrigeration
refrigeration and eating.

3. Watch environment
Clean well and disinfect
Keep apart raw and cooked foods.

Appendix B

PREVENTION OF FOOD POISONING ABROAD

Most people travelling in Europe, Asia, the Far East, South America and Africa experience gastro-enteritis. Some accept it as inevitable and include in their luggage prophylactic and treatment pills and medicines of various kinds.

It follows meals eaten on intercontinental ships, trains and planes, in hotels, boarding houses and private houses and during camping from food bought in local shops and markets.

The patterns of illness follow those described in the previous chapters and all types of bacterial food poisoning are encountered.

There is much so-called non-specific diarrhoea or 'gippy-tummy' which is said to be due to change of food, overeating, overdrinking, heat, rapid change of temperature, iced drinks and so on. Unfortunately, the facilities for a full and competent investigation of these illnesses are rarely available. Bacteriological laboratories are not carried routinely, even in the largest and most important shipping lines, nor, of course, on trains.

The traveller on land accepts his predicament knowing that he will soon recover; when medical aid is summoned the doctor recognizes the well known symptoms and seeks to relieve the condition without taking time to study the cause.

While allowing for the fact that loose stools are likely to occur sometimes during a holiday overseas, due to strange foods and cooking habits, and to overdoses of aperients following constipation, the vast majority of incidents are likely to be microbial in origin. The principles underlying the provision of safe food are the same by whatever means one chooses to travel and in whatever country one chooses to be. The countries with hot climates will have greater problems than those in the north; refrigerators are a necessity where it is consistently hot, whereas temperate countries may require refrigeration as a luxury instead of necessity. Particular food habits in certain countries may expose the inhabitants and the travellers to special hazards. For example, the eating of raw fermented fish dishes in the Arctic and Japan has given rise to botulism and, in Japan, to much food poisoning caused by *Vibrio parahaemolyticus*. The recognition of this type of food poisoning is growing in countries other than Japan and the importance of cross contamination from raw to cooked seafoods has been reported. On the other hand care in the processing of canned foods, a distaste for raw fish and general habits of home preservation which include heat treatment of acid fruits but rarely meat, poultry, game or vegetables have no doubt protected the population of the British Isles from botulism. This fatal food poisoning occurs frequently in countries where housewives cure and heat preserve many foods. The prevalence of *Clostridium welchii* food poisoning in England and Wales may be related to the habit of precooking and warming meat dishes, a practice which became more prevalent in the war years due to shortage of meat.

Rules for travellers

1. Avoid drinking or cleaning teeth in cold water unless it has been either personally chlorinated by the addition of proprietary brands of tablets or liquids containing sodium hypochlorite, or pumped through a filter such as the Berkefeld filter. Wines, bottled mineral water and soft drinks are safe.

2. Avoid using ice in drinks as the ice may be prepared from impure water

3. Foods to be avoided unless their safety is guaranteed:
   (a) Ice-cream, as few countries outside the United Kingdom have legislation governing the method of production, which can be subject to many faults in hygiene.
   (b) Milk, unless pasteurized or boiled, and any form of fermented milk.
   (c) Soft and semi-hard cheese, particularly goats' milk cheese. In many Continental countries soft cheeses are prepared from pasteurized or boiled milk and are safe; this may or may not be stated on the packet. In the Middle or Far East such cheese is usually prepared from raw or inadequately heated milk and may be bacteriologically dangerous.
   (d) Cooked or semi-preserved cold meats, sausages and meat sandwiches, which may be subjected to much handling and poor storage in warm countries; with the exception of those products known to have a very high salt content.
   (e) Meatballs, which are popular in some countries and may be

prepared with meat cooked ahead of requirements and thus be a suitable medium for the growth of *Cl. welchii.*

(f) Curried foods prepared some hours before required and kept warm pending consumption.

(g) Shell-fish and other seafoods, particularly from warm countries.

(h) 'Bar tasties', particularly those including prawns and other seafoods.

(i) Cooked chickens, unless seen to be freshly cooked in a reputable shop.

(j) Salads and dessert fruits, unless carefully washed in water containing hypochlorite.

Campers and travellers who buy their own picnic lunches can take care of their own purchases and preparation of food. Meals eaten out at night should be chosen with regard to freshly cooked meat, e.g. grills and fresh roasts.

Those who live in tents, caravans and cars should take precautions with tea towels and dish cloths which should be washed thoroughly and stored in or wrung out in disinfectant after use. However, preferably disposable paper instead of cloths should be used. A similar precaution applies to flannels. Children are particularly susceptible to gastro-enteritis and as a precaution against infection from hands each child should rinse the hands in disinfectant before and after meals. This practice should apply also to adults preparing food.

The floor of caravans should be washed over daily with disinfectant.

A list of names of suitable disinfectants should be available from the local medical officer of health or chief public health inspector.

It may be considered by some that the precautions are unnecessary and troublesome to carry out; the alternative may be at best a short attack of gastro-enteritis or at the worst an attack of typhoid or paratyphoid fever or dysentery during the holiday or after returning home. However, holidays may be expensive and it is a pity to lose days by illness.

It may be reasoned that similar precautions should be taken in the home country and this is true, but when crowds in holiday countries must be fed quickly and atmospheric temperatures are soaring, the hazards of mass feeding are magnified.

Index